OPTIMAL MUSCLE TRAINING

Ken Kinakin

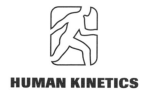

HUMAN KINETICS

Library of Congress Cataloging-in-Publication Data

Kinakin, Ken., 1962-
    Optimal muscle training / Ken Kinakin.
        p. cm.
Includes bibliographical references and index.
    ISBN 0-7360-4679-8 (hard cover)
    1. Muscle strength. 2. Weight training. I. Title.
    QP321.K49 2003
    613.7'1--dc22

                                                            2003014322
ISBN: 0-7360-4679-8

Acquisitions Editor: Edward McNeely; **Developmental Editor:** Anne Cole; **Assistant Editors:** Scott Hawkins and Kim Thoren; **Copyeditor:** Karen Bojda; **Proofreader:** Kathy Bennett; **Indexer:** Craig Brown; **Permissions Manager:** Toni Harte; **Graphic Designer:** Robert Reuther; **Graphic Artist:** Francine Hamerski; **Art and Photo Manager:** Dan Wendt; **Cover Designer:** Keith Blomberg; **Photographer (cover):** Dan Wendt; **Photographer (interior):** Ken Kinakin; **Illustrator:** © Eric Blais www.ericblaisart.com; **Printer:** Imprelibros S. A.

Human Kinetics books are available at special discounts for bulk purchase. Special editions or book excerpts can also be created to specification. For details, contact the Special Sales Manager at Human Kinetics.

Printed in Colombia 10 9 8 7 6 5 4 3 2 1

Human Kinetics
Web site: www.HumanKinetics.com

United States: Human Kinetics
P.O. Box 5076
Champaign, IL 61825-5076
800-747-4457
e-mail: humank@hkusa.com

Canada: Human Kinetics
475 Devonshire Road Unit 100
Windsor, ON N8Y 2L5
800-465-7301 (in Canada only)
e-mail: orders@hkcanada.com

Europe: Human Kinetics
107 Bradford Road
Stanningley
Leeds LS28 6AT, United Kingdom
+44 (0) 113 255 5665
e-mail: hk@hkeurope.com

Australia: Human Kinetics
57A Price Avenue
Lower Mitcham, South Australia 5062
08 8277 1555
e-mail: liaw@hkaustralia.com

New Zealand: Human Kinetics
Division of Sports Distributors NZ Ltd.
P.O. Box 300 226 Albany
North Shore City
Auckland
0064 9 448 1207
e-mail: blairc@hknewz.com

OPTIMAL
MUSCLE
TRAINING

Contents

Product Features

Welcome to *Optimal Muscle Training,* a unique book and DVD package presenting the keys to optimizing muscle, joint, nerve, and biochemical functions and mastering the technical aspects of resistance exercises.

The book provides the background information necessary to optimize your potential for strength and muscle development. It explains how muscles function, provides tests to determine your ability to do specific weight-training exercises, and discusses the exercises that are most beneficial for various training outcomes and goals. The final chapter offers the road map to improved functional level and optimized performance.

The enclosed DVD walks you through the weight-training readiness tests, demonstrates proper technique for specific weight-training exercises, and offers forms and scoring sheets. It features video demonstrations of 33 weight-training exercises; 136 tests for weight-training readiness; and 70 flexibility, isometric, PNF, and tubing exercises. The forms and scoring sheets will assist you in testing and analyzing your ability to train effectively. You can view the video content either on a television set with a DVD player or on a computer with a DVD-ROM drive. The forms and scoring sheets can only be accessed through the DVD-ROM drive on your computer (see the instructions at the end of this section).

The DVD is divided into 10 sections, each representing a body part, so that you can focus separately on training the shoulders, chest, upper back, lower back, triceps, biceps, forearms, abdominals, legs, and calves. For each section, a menu with three buttons allows you to choose Optimal Technique, Assessment, and Functional Training for that body part. All menus on the DVD allow you to return to the Main Menu and to navigate quickly within each section.

Under Optimal Technique, you will see demonstrations of basic strength-training exercises and hear a narration that describes proper technique. You can use these techniques to improve your own training or you can use it with clients, team members, and friends.

The Assessment sections are divided into three types of testing: the self-test, the functional muscle test, and the exercise test. The self-test contains several movements that test, without weights, your ability to move with proper technique through the full range of motion. You can use the scoring sheets on the DVD-ROM to rate your performance. After each self-test, the DVD will route you to the next test if you have full range of motion and no pain, or to functional training exercises if you experienced decreased range of motion or pain.

The functional muscle test demonstrates how fitness professionals, therapists, and physicians can test their clients' weight-training readiness and determine functional weaknesses. This is an excellent section for professional trainers to use for testing muscle performance in each exercise.

The exercise test presents strength-training exercises and reviews the optimal techniques for each. Then it describes and demonstrates common problems caused by weaknesses and dysfunctions in the muscles, joints, or nerves that are being trained. This section also uses a scoring system that guides you to functional training exercises if any pain or weaknesses exist.

The Functional Training sections guide you to supplementary flexibility, isometric, and tubing exercises using the muscles worked in the strength-training exercises for each body area. PNF exercises are also included for the chest, shoulders, and upper back. You can navigate to these exercises by identifying the muscle that needs work and then selecting the Supplemental Exercise button for each major weight-training exercise.

How to Use the DVD

To use the DVD, place it in your DVD player or DVD-ROM drive. A title screen will welcome you to the program. Then the Main Menu with buttons for each body area will appear. When you click on one of the buttons for a body area, you will have a choice of viewing Optimal Technique, Assessment, or Functional Training. Once you've navigated into each of these three areas, you will be able to retrace your steps by using the Back button on the bottom of each page. Or, you can return to the overall list of body areas by using the Main Menu button. When buttons on the bottom row are highlighted, you can move from Optimal Technique to Assessment by selecting the appropriate button.

To access the forms and scoring sheets from Windows®,

1. Insert the DVD into your DVD-ROM drive.
2. Access Windows® Explorer.
3. Click on the DVD-ROM drive icon.
4. Select the PDF file you want to view.

To access the forms and scoring sheets on a Macintosh® computer,

1. Insert the DVD into your DVD-ROM drive.
2. Double-click on the "Optimal Muscle Training" DVD icon on your desktop.
3. Select the PDF file you want to view.

Note: If your DVD viewing program is set to automatically launch, the video content will automatically run. You will need to close out of the DVD viewing program before accessing the PDF files.

The PDF files can only be accessed through the DVD-ROM drive on your computer. If you do not have a DVD-ROM drive on your computer, the Web site www.optimalmuscletraining.com contains the forms as well as other information. You will not be able to access these forms on your television.

You will need Adobe® Reader® to view the PDF files. If you do not already have Adobe Reader installed on your computer, go to www.adobe.com to download the free software.

Select the HK Running Man logo on the Main Menu to access production credits and information on contacting Human Kinetics to order other products.

Preface

This book was written to educate trainers, doctors, therapists, and weight-training enthusiasts about optimizing muscle function during weight training. At the heart of this book is a simple process: assessing functional level and then finding out how to use weight training to optimize a person's full potential. Each person's unique biomechanics and functional status affects his or her weight-training program. These issues need to be addressed logically, step by step, to design an optimal weight-training program.

The weight-training readiness exam described in this book and demonstrated on the DVD includes three different types of assessment: a self-test, an exercise test, and a functional muscle test. The self-test determines the pain-free range of motion for weight-training exercises. The exercise test determines whether the athlete has pain-free symmetrical strength while doing various weight-training exercises. The functional muscle test is administered by a doctor, therapist, or trainer and uses advanced muscle-testing procedures to assess nerve, joint, and muscle function and determine whether the person has any pain or weakness while weight training. These tests assess the state of the person's body to determine his or her level of functionality. The results of these tests help determine the optimal weight-training exercises for each person's biomechanics to decrease risk of injury while maximizing strength and performance.

To design an optimal weight-training program, it is also important to understand functional anatomy: where muscles attach and how they function in the body. This information helps you understand how specific techniques can increase the effectiveness of exercises and also the risks and benefits of performing them. The program design process presented in the last chapter takes into consideration individual limitations, biomechanics, and desired training outcomes and goals.

If this book and DVD can help you achieve your full potential, then their goal in being developed will be accomplished.

Acknowledgments

If I have seen further, it is by standing on the shoulders of giants.
—Sir Isaac Newton, February 5, 1675

In my two decades of health and fitness experience I have met many giants who are innovators and mentors, and I am honored to say many of them are my friends. The giants in the training, treatment, and nutrition fields that have contributed their concepts to this book are Dr. David Leaf, Dr. Mike Leahy, Dr. Mauro Di Pasquale, Dr. Mark Lindsay, Dr. Eric Serrano, Dr. Alexander Wood, Bill Pearl, Matt Nichol, Dr. Mark Percival, Dr. Dale Buchberger, Dr. Mike Hartle, Charles Poliquin, Dr. Dave Harper, Dr. Geron Cowherd, Lorne Goldenberg, Paul Chek, Dr. Rob Rakowski, Dr. Alejandro Elorriaga, Dr. Mark Scappaticci, Dr. George Gonzalez, Dr. Richard Amy, Dr. Guy Voyer, Scott Abel, Dr. John Berardi, Ian King, Dr. Dan Kirsch, Dr. George Goodheart, Dr. Barry Sears, Dr. Tom Deters, Laura Binetti, Dr. Mel Siff, Ed Coan, Lee Haney, Dave Tate, Louie Simmons, Rickey Dale Crain, Milos Sarcev, Mohamed Makkawy, Laura Creavalle, Winston Roberts, Harvey Newton, Chad Ikei, David Sandler, Mark Verstegan, Brian Johnston, Dr. Jeff Spencer, Peter Twist, Kate Pace Lindsay, Doug Caporrino, Dr. Mark Charrette, Dr. George Roth, Dr. Dan Murphy, Greg Roskopf, Ann and Chris Frederick, Dr. Fred Kahn, Dr. Sylvain Guimond, Dr. James Oschman, Dr. Jerome Rerucha, Dr. Carl DeRosa, Dr. Chris Colloca, Paul Gagne, Dr. Michele Joubert, Dr. Udo Erasmus, Dr. Lonnie Lowery, Dorian Yates, Dr. Steve Segal, Ming Chew, Aaron Mattes, Sheldon Persad, Barrie Shepley, Dr. Alain Vaillancourt, Dr. Tom Bilella, Bill Kazmaier, Charlie Francis, Istvan Balyi, Charles Staley, Dr. Stuart McGill, Dr. Jacek Cholewicki, Dr. Duncan McDougall, Dr. Digby Sale, and Dr. Jim Nichols.

The people at Human Kinetics have been amazing in their work on this book and DVD. I would like to personally thank Ed McNeely, Doug Fink, Brian Stumph, Anne Cole, Coree Clark, Roger Francisco, Chris Clark, Mark Herman, Amy Rose, and Mike Bates.

I am indebted to Jack Kinakin, Simone Lewis, John Foulkes, and Yvette Patai, the exercise models who helped make this an excellent product. Eric Blais created beautiful artwork that illustrates the various types of dysfunctions that may occur from training.

I would like to personally thank Heidi Hess, Stephanie Anisko, Jenny Candido, Emily North, Keri Feldman, and Sabrina Daniels, the staff members of SWIS and my clinic who have been very supportive throughout the last year of writing the book and DVD. Thank you.

I thank my friends who have helped me in so many ways throughout this book's writing process: Mike Milanovic, Lucinda Christian, Dr. Markus Thiel, Jen Thiel, Rory Mullin, Alana and Craig Aird, Jon Soyka, Josie Casale, Gil Ansah, Andy Belanger, Vera Bond, Libby Norris, Richard Lefebvre, Frances Michaelson, Sylvie Duval, Carolyn Little, Dr. Ward Hazen, Dr. Dawn Cormier, John and Gerda Heffener, Steve Hunter, Matt Jones, Dr. Larry Kinakin, Susan Lee, Dr. Jan Lichti, Lori MacIntyre, Mike Ettles, Dore Blais, Cheri Percival, Dr. Greg MacLuckie, Katrina Newell, Kim and Irene Piller, Lynn Perry, Dr. Doug Price, Dr. Keith Pyne, Sam Rodrigues, Myles Mana, Brendan Regan, Jim Smith, Darryl Williamson, and Anthony Robbins.

This book and DVD are dedicated to my parents, Bill and Virginia Kinakin, and my brother and sister, Jack Kinakin and Karen Liscia. They have all been so supportive over the years with all my wild ideas and dreams of becoming a doctor of chiropractic and also organizing massive SWIS symposiums where I invited the best in the world to learn, share, and revolutionize the health and fitness industry. This book and DVD arose from those dreams and events. Thank you, everyone, for making my dreams come true.

1

The Anatomy of Optimizing Strength

The main focus of any weight-training routine is to optimize your potential for strength and development. Many things can create what is known as a weight-training dysfunction that can limit lifting potential. A weight-training dysfunction is an abnormality in a structure or system that causes an alteration in how the body performs during weight training. Weight-training dysfunctions can develop from a variety of sources, such as poor lifting technique, lifting beyond one's capabilities, training too often, and insufficient rest or recuperation. An often-overlooked cause is a previously injured area that does not heal correctly and becomes dysfunctional when an excessive load is put on it.

To prevent weight-training dysfunctions most effectively, three different approaches should be taken. The first approach is to use excellent lifting technique. The second is to make sure that the exercises performed are not contraindicated for biomechanical reasons. The third is to test to make sure that muscles, joints, nerves, and biochemistry are all working optimally and have no dysfunction.

Four Types of Weight-Training Dysfunction

A weight-training dysfunction is much different than an injury in a contact sport such as hockey or football and from an overuse injury in an activity such as running. Weight-training dysfunctions can be caused by a lack of recuperation that causes microtrauma (small amounts of muscle damage important for growth and strength) to develop into macrotrauma (a large amount of damage that does not contribute to muscle growth or strength but instead actually prevents training due to pain). Macrotrauma can affect muscle, joint, or nerve or create a biochemical problem and is the usual cause of weight-training injuries. One or more of these types of injuries can be present at the same time, causing pain, weakness, and altered joint motion during an exercise. The more complex and chronic the problem, the more likely that multiple types of dysfunction are going on at the same time.

Four types of weight-training dysfunctions can occur:

1. Muscle dysfunction occurs when muscle has been damaged and has scar tissue, a muscle imbalance exists, the muscle is shortened, or the muscle is deconditioned.

2. Joint dysfunction occurs when there is abnormal motion of a joint, the joint is compressed, or a joint has become separated.

3. Nerve dysfunction occurs when tension or compression of the nerve has decreased or altered the action potentials of the nerve. Altered proprioception at the joint can inhibit the potential strength of the muscle also.

4. Biochemical dysfunction occurs when overtraining or deficiency in specific nutrients causes a global lack of strength and recovery that can contribute to the chronicity of the injury.

Muscle Dysfunction

The first factor in dysfunction is muscle damage that causes pain and weakness. If the muscle is damaged, it usually has some inflammation. If the inflammation is mild enough, it tends to go away in a few days or weeks. More extensive muscular damage causes macrotrauma. The body responds to this by forming adhesions, or scar tissue (figure 1.1), between the sheaths, or fascia, of adjacent fiber bundles in the muscle (Akeson and Amiel 1977; Barnes 1997; Donatelli 1981). These fibrous adhesions limit the ease and range of motion of muscles and joints and can decrease the muscles' lengthening and shortening capabilities. Once the normal biomechanics of a joint is altered, further inflammation can ensue, instigating a vicious cycle of long-term wear and tear.

This fibrous adhesion pattern can be seen in people who do exercises such as the bench press and complain of the same pain in the exact same spot. This pain does not recur by chance. A fibrous adhesion formed in the shoulder muscle can prevent proper movement and pull on the various soft-tissue structures, such as the muscle, fascia, tendon, and bursa, when performing the bench press.

Taking time off from lifting will decrease the chronic inflammation, but it will not decrease the fibrous adhesion. As soon as training starts again, the fibrous adhesion will restrict proper motion and again cause pain that prevents performance of this exercise. An analogy is when your car tire shakes while driving. Putting the car in the garage for one month and not driving it will prevent further damage to the tire and steering linkages, but it will not fix the tire alignment. You have to take it to a mechanic who can properly assess the altered tire alignment and then balance the tire until it spins perfectly again. Similarly, with an injury, all the possible fibrous adhesions in the muscle must be identified, and then some soft-tissue therapy must be performed to break up all those fibrous adhesions in the muscle, muscle sheaths, tendons, ligaments, and fascia.

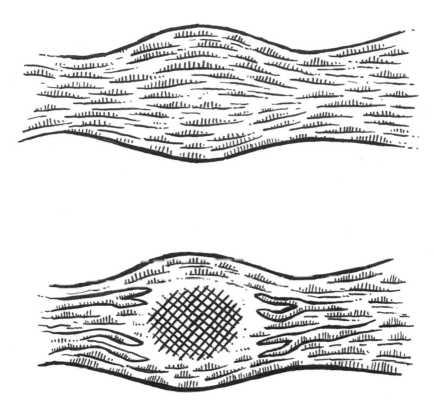

Figure 1.1 Normal muscle tissue *(top);* scar tissue and fibrous adhesions within the muscle *(bottom).*

Another type of muscle dysfunction is the trigger point (a tender, localized hardening) in a muscle, which can inhibit other muscles. Simon (1993) reported that the deltoid muscle can be inhibited during shoulder flexion when the infraspinatus muscle has trigger points. Headley (1993) also found inhibition of the lower trapezius muscle during shoulder flexion and abduction when there are trigger points in the upper trapezius. Soft-tissue treatment on trigger points is needed to restore normal muscular function.

Joint Dysfunction

Another area that can contribute to a weight-training dysfunction is the joint that the muscle crosses. If the trauma is mild enough, a muscle dysfunction can exist without affecting the joint directly. However, if the joint is traumatized, the muscle, tendon, and ligaments are also usually injured because of the excessive amount of force experienced on the stabilizing structures of the joint.

Most weight-training joint dysfunctions can be classified in two categories: compression injuries and tearing injuries. These injuries can be either mild, moderate, or severe and can take days, weeks, and sometimes even months to heal, depending on their severity and how aggressively treatment is pursued.

Weight-Training Compression Injury

In a weight-training compression injury, trauma usually occurs at the joint itself. This type of injury involves little or no tearing of the tissues. Swelling, if any, is limited to the joint capsule. Excessive stress and load in weight training affects mechanoreceptors and nociceptors (small receptors in the joint that give the body information about position, load, and pain) in the joint structure (Walther 1988; Norris 2000). This type of injury appears to affect the internal structures of the joint and commonly causes weakness in multiple muscles, especially muscles that cross the joint. Joints that can be affected by weight-training compression injuries are the ankle, the knee, and the lumbar, thoracic, and cervical vertebrae (figure 1.2). The exercises that can affect these joints are usually those with a heavy downward pressure on the spine (for example, heavy squats, dead lifts, and standing shoulder presses). These heavy loads can compress the joints enough to create abnormal firing of joint receptors and can change the normal tone and strength of the muscles that surround the joint.

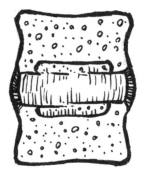 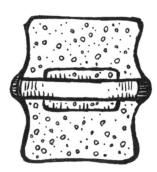

Figure 1.2   Normal vertebra and disc *(left)*; severe compression of vertebral disc *(right)*.

Weight-Training Tearing Injury

A weight-training tearing injury (figure 1.3) can affect multiple structures. This is the most common type of joint injury and occurs when joints and related structures are strained and twisted, injuring muscles, tendons, ligaments, and cartilage of the joints. Any joint in the body can be affected by a tearing injury, and a tearing injury can be caused by almost any exercise (Woo and Buckwalter 1988).

A weight-training tearing injury can cause inflammation and weakness of the muscles that cross the joint. When the joints become inflamed, there is a reflex inhibition of the muscles that cross that joint (DeAndrade, Grant, and Doxon 1965; Spencer, Hayes, and Alexander 1984). Ligaments are structures that cross and stabilize the joint and, when stressed abnormally, can also cause abnormal function in the muscles that cross the joint (Johansson and Sjolander 1990). Certain receptors in ligaments, when overloaded, cause a reflex contracture of the muscle, thus shortening it and causing potential muscle weakness (Solomonow 1998). This is a protective mechanism to prevent instability and further damage to the joint.

Depending on the severity of the injury and the length of time before initiation of treatment, the injured person will adapt to the injury and require treatment for

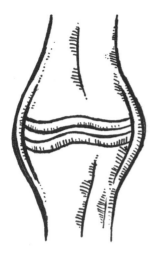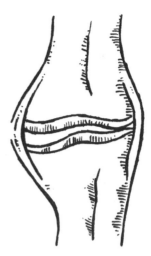

Figure 1.3 Normal knee (left); severe knee tearing injury *(right)*.

muscle imbalance. This imbalance brings about secondary pain and weakness in the muscle when exercising long after the initial injury. Limited range of motion can indicate an imbalance of the prime movers and the synergistic or supportive muscles. For example, doing a squat improperly can injure the knee. This injury causes abnormal stress on the knee ligaments and results in weakness of the muscles that cross the knee joint, such as the quadriceps and hamstrings. Failure to treat and rehabilitate the knee injury properly can cause an imbalance between the quadriceps and hamstrings, in turn creating more pain and weakness. If the imbalance is severe enough or persists long enough, it can also cause stress in other joints and weakness in other muscles unrelated to the original injury, which in turn can affect training and can hamper gains.

Nerve Dysfunction

A nerve that is either stretched (figure 1.4) or compressed can have a major effect on the strength of the muscle it innervates (supplies). The best example of this is sleeping all night with your arm above your head. In the morning, if the phone rings and you try to pick it up, you notice that your arm cannot move. It has fallen asleep, and you have to pick it up with your other hand and shake it out until feeling returns with a pins and needles sensation. Only then do you have enough strength to pick up the phone.

The same dysfunction can occur in weight training. An example is pushing too hard in a back workout and overstressing the lumbar spine. During the next day's leg workout, the right leg may seem weaker than the left during squats, and the lifter may twist the trunk while coming out of the bottom of the exercise. Strength is less than usual and the lifter may have a hard time with weights that normally seem light. The lifter may think nothing of it and just feel that some time is needed to recover. But next week, the lifter may notice pain in the right knee when doing a leg press, and strength still may not have returned to normal. One week after

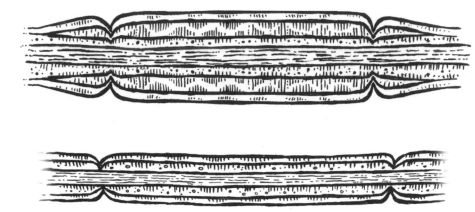

Figure 1.4 Normal nerve *(top)*; nerve under tension *(bottom)*.

that, the leg is still weaker than usual. Strength in all the leg exercises is affected, and the lifter is starting to feel more pain in the right knee and hip. At this point, a week off may sometimes work to relieve the pain and regain strength, but as soon as the lifter works out with heavier weights, the weakness returns and pain is not far behind.

What happened? Research over the past few years has given us some insight that is rarely discussed or presented with regard to weight training. Some studies have shown that decreasing the nerve supply to muscles can reduce strength and create a possible scenario for pain. If the nerves from the spine to the muscles undergo any compression or, more commonly, any tension, the decreased nerve supply causes a decline in performance and increased risk of injury if heavier weights are used. Research reveals that only a small amount of compression or tension is needed to create this type of weakness. Rydevik (1991) reported that compression of only 10 to 50 millimeters of mercury (the weight of a dime on the back of your hand) can potentially decrease action potentials by up to 40 percent. MacNab (1972) found that compression without pain can cause a neurological deficit or weakness. Wall (1992) found that a 6 percent strain (tension) decreased action potentials by over 70 percent. This is why taking time off from training without addressing the underlying cause of the problem will not work; as soon as heavy weights are used again, the problems come back. With any injury it is imperative that the muscles, joints, and nerves be examined to find out what is causing the pain and weakness and that all causes be treated at the same time.

Biochemical Dysfunction

Biochemical dysfunction is becoming more common but is rarely discussed. Overtraining or deficiency in specific nutrients can cause a global decrease of strength that can contribute to chronic injury. Chronic stress due to overtraining impairs normal adrenal production, causing pain, weakness, and the inability to respond to stress of any kind. It can take weeks or months to recover from these detrimental effects of stress. A nutrient deficiency can result from an extremely strict diet in which the same few foods are eaten every day. This is seen especially in competitive bodybuilders, whose diet is often high in protein with minimal amounts of vegetables and who thus receive less than optimal amounts of vitamins and minerals. Their adrenal glands are overstressed by not having enough nutrients to handle the increased work demand of heavy weights and strenuous cardio work.

Chronic stress or overtraining can create a condition called relative adrenal insufficiency, in which the adrenal glands fail to produce an adequate amount of secretions for the body to function optimally for the relative amount of stress experienced. This condition is different from a clinical disease, such as Addison's or Cushing's disease, that is caused by pathology. The status of an individual doing heavy training may fall somewhere in between optimal function and disease pathology. The adrenal gland produces secretions via two hormonal pathways during hard training: epinephrine and norepinephrine from the adrenal medulla and cortisol and testosterone from the adrenal cortex. Epinephrine is released when a known or expected stressor, such as training, stresses the body. The adrenal medulla needs protein and the cofactors tyrosine and niacin for proper production of epinephrine. Norepinephrine is released in response to unexpected or unknown stressors, as in a fight or flight situation. The production of norepinephrine depends on levels of cholesterol and the cofactors vitamin C, vitamin B_6, niacin, folic acid, and pantothenic acid in the body. Without optimal amounts of cofactors, the adrenal medulla cannot produce enough epinephrine and norepinephrine. If these hormones are not at optimal levels, a person may have difficulty responding to heavy training. The body may begin to break down and have a greater potential to be injured. Due to insufficient protein in their diets, vegetarians and women may have less of these hormones than men who usually have a higher amount of protein in their diet.

The production of cortisol and testosterone from the adrenal cortex depends on levels of cholesterol and the cofactors vitamin C, pantothenic acid, vitamin B_6, niacinamide, zinc, and folic acid. A deficiency in these hormones decreases the ability to handle heavy training and the lifter may experience an increased amount of pain.

Causes of Weight-Training Dysfunction

Weight-training dysfunctions can develop from a variety of sources:

- Poor lifting technique. Poor lifting technique usually results from a lack of direct supervision and lack of attention to lifting biomechanics. On the DVD, proper technique and form are presented, along with abnormal technique caused by dysfunction.

- Lifting beyond one's capabilities. Training with heavier loads increases the possibility of tissue and structure failure due to either poor conditioning of the soft-tissue structures or neurological fatigue, which both contribute to poor technique.

- Training too often. When a muscle has been exercised, it needs time to recover from the stress of training so that it can hypertrophy. If you train the same body part too frequently, it doesn't have time to recover properly, increasing inflammation and scar tissue in the area.

■ Insufficient rest or recuperation. Not resting properly between training sessions makes it difficult to train heavily at the next session. Outside stressors of life can also affect recuperation, and everything possible should be done to minimize those stressors.

■ Performing the same exercises on machines all the time. Training in the same plane and range of motion on a machine all the time can create dysfunctions within the muscle being worked. Paton and Brown (1994) described a concept called functional differentiation, which suggests that when a muscle with a broad origin, such as the pectoral muscle, is exercised, the central nervous system fine-tunes the activation pattern to maximally contract only a segment of that muscle. Thus, always training on the same machines can create a strength disparity within the same muscle group. The way to prevent this is to use a variety of machines and free weights.

■ Previously injured areas that did not heal correctly. One of the main causes of weight-training dysfunction is a previous injury that did not heal properly and is exposed by overloading the joint or muscle. This is commonly seen when only one side is injured during heavy training. It has been hypothesized that weight training, rather than causing injuries, often exposes previous injuries that were never treated and rehabilitated properly. If an exercise performed with both arms or legs truly was the cause of an injury, the injury would occur on both sides since the same amount of weight is handled on both arms or both legs.

Assessment of Weight-Training Function

Three questionnaires can help assess weight-training function and determine whether any of the four weight-training dysfunctions are present.

The Weight-Training Readiness Screen (see page 10) helps determine whether any problems or pain occur during training. It doesn't determine the cause, only whether there is a problem. The Weight-Training Readiness Form (see page 15) determines the dysfunctional area and helps differentiate muscle, joint, and nerve problems. The Subjective Training Stress Level Questionnaire (see page 16) determines whether any symptoms are related to a biochemical dysfunction.

These forms determine whether an exam by a doctor or therapist is needed. If so, the doctor or therapist can determine the extent of the dysfunction and whether specific treatment and exercises are appropriate.

Weight-Training Readiness Screen

This questionnaire reveals whether there is any pain while weight training and whether the athlete is modifying his or her routine by avoiding certain exercises or body parts. Each answer is associated with a number to quantify the severity of the dysfunction. To score, add these numbers up and circle the total on the scoring scale. The total score is used to determine the remedial action needed.

This screen includes five questions about weight-training dysfunctions:

1. Do you have pain while weight training?

This straightforward question determines whether a dysfunction is severe enough to cause pain. It is important to note that absence of pain does not mean that there is no problem. In addition, people have varied perceptions of pain and may overstate or understate its significance.

2. Do you avoid certain exercises that you used to do or avoid exercising certain body parts because of pain or difficulty doing those exercises?

This is one of the most important questions in the screen. It determines whether there is a problem with weight-training technique or with a muscle, joint, or nerve. Four different levels of function are possible:

a. Can perform any exercise for any body part pain-free with full strength.

b. Avoid one specific exercise due to pain or weakness. This means that the exercise was deleted from the routine due to difficulty performing it and pain or weakness. If this is the case, review weight-training technique to determine if poor technique is causing pain. If technique is good, assess the body to determine what dysfunction is causing the pain or weakness.

c. Avoid more than one exercise for a body part due to pain or weakness. When many exercises for the same body part cause pain or weakness, check weight-training technique and fill out the Weight-Training Readiness Form (see page 15) to determine if there is a muscle, joint, or nerve problem.

d. Avoid training an entire body part due to pain or weakness. The body part causes pain even when exercising other muscle groups, for example, when the shoulders are painful while training the chest or arms. In this case, check weight-training technique, fill out the Weight-Training Readiness Form (see page 15) to determine if there is a muscle, joint, or nerve problem. Then do a Weight-Training Readiness Exam (see page 19) to further assess the problem and determine the appropriate exercises or treatment needed to help restore normal function.

For a printable version of the forms in this chapter, access the forms on the DVD.

3. If you are experiencing a problem, how long have you had it?

This answer quickly ascertains whether any dysfunction is acute and recent (days or weeks) or chronic and long-standing (months or years). When the problem is chronic, a compensation pattern maybe developing where other muscles or joints are being affected.

4. Do you feel your body compensating when exercising, as by one arm lagging behind when pressing or your body twisting when squatting?

These classic signs of weight-training dysfunction reveal that something is wrong with either the muscle, joint, or nerve. Both limbs should have the same strength when doing any exercise. Any deviation is a sign that something is not

Weight-Training Readiness Screen

Name: _____

Date: _____

Part A: Questionnaire

Please check the boxes that best apply right now.

1. Do you have pain while weight training?

   ❑ No (0)　　　❑ Mild (1)　　　❑ Moderate (2)　　❑ Severe (3)

2. Do you avoid certain exercises that you used to do or avoid exercising certain body parts because of pain or difficulty doing those exercises?

   ❑ No (0) Can perform any exercise for any body part pain-free with full strength.

   ❑ Yes (select a response below)

   ❑ Avoid one specific exercise due to pain or weakness (score 1 point)

   Which exercise? _____

   ❑ Avoid more than one exercise for a body part due to pain or weakness (score 2 points)

   Which exercises? _____

   ❑ Avoid training an entire body part due to pain or weakness (score 3 points)

   Which body part? _____

3. If you are experiencing a problem, how long have you had it?

   ❑ No problem (0)　　　❑ Days (1)　　　❑ Weeks (2)　　❑ Months (3)

4. Do you feel your body compensating when exercising, as by one arm lagging behind when bench pressing or your body twisting when squatting?

   ❑ No (0)　　　❑ Mildly (1)　　　❑ Moderately (2)　　❑ Severely (3)

5. Have you felt a strength decrease in specific exercises?

   ❑ No (0)　　　❑ Mild (1)　　　❑ Moderate (2)　　❑ Severe (3)

Part B: Score

Add up the numbers that correspond to the checked boxes, and circle the corresponding number below.

0　1　2　3　4　5　6　7　8　9　10　11　12　13　14　15
　None　　　　　　Mild　　　　　　Moderate　　　　　　Severe

Part C: Interpretation

Total Score

0   No problems. Keep training.

1–5   Check weight-training technique. Monitor the body area and exercise to see whether the problem gets worse. The Weight-Training Readiness Exam (see description in chapter 2 on page 19) may be beneficial to evaluate for any hidden problems.

6–10   Check weight-training technique. The Weight-Training Readiness Exam (see description in chapter 2 on page 19) is **advised** to prevent further damage.

11–15   Check weight-training technique. The Weight-Training Readiness Exam (see description in chapter 2 on page 19) is **required** to assess the dysfunction to prevent further damage.

Question 2

0   No problems. Keep training.

1   Check weight-training technique to determine whether poor technique is causing pain or weakness.

2   Check weight training technique. Fill out the Weight-Training Readiness Form for further investigation on the dysfunction.

3   Check weight-training technique. Fill out the Weight-Training Readiness Form and perform the Weight-Training Readiness Exam (see description in chapter 2 on page 19).

Part D: Comments and Action

❏   No problems; continue training.

❏   Fill out the Weight-Training Readiness Form for further investigation.

❏   Set up appointment for the Weight-Training Readiness Exam (see description in chapter 2 on page 19) to assess severity of problem.

❏   Set up appointment with doctor or therapist for further investigation.

Comments:

working correctly. Specific exercises may be needed to strengthen the area, but first it must be determined whether the problem is with the muscle, joint, or nerve. It can be very difficult to strengthen a dysfunctional muscle, joint, or nerve with weight-training exercises alone. It may need specific rehabilitation exercises or treatment first, then strengthening with weight-training exercises.

5. Have you felt a strength decrease in specific exercises?

Weakness is usually an indicator that something is wrong and that it is getting worse. If an area becomes dysfunctional, first it starts to lose strength. If training continues, the area may become weaker and also start to have pain. This is the body's way to protect itself from further damage. The affected area needs to be checked for a muscle, joint, or nerve dysfunction, and specific rehabilitative exercises or treatment may be needed to restore normal function.

Scoring and Interpretation

1. Add up the numbers that correspond to the answers checked, and circle the total on the scale in part B. This provides a visual indicator of the severity of the problem.

2. Find the total score in part C, and review what needs to be done.

3. Find the score for just question 2 in the section "Question 2 Interpretation" in part C, and review what needs to be done.

4. In part D, check the appropriate box based on the scoring, and review what needs to be done.

Weight-Training Readiness Form

The Weight-Training Readiness Form enables the doctor, therapist, or trainer to analyze a weight-training dysfunction and how it affects training. The results identify exercises that cause pain; the effectiveness of training or treatment can be measured by reduced pain and increased strength. Isolating the exercises and motions that cause the pain also helps identify the specific muscles or joints that may need rehabilitative training or treatment and provides information about which exercises to refrain from temporarily.

A personal trainer can also use the form to decide whether to refer the person to a doctor or therapist for treatment. Tingling or numbness revealed by the form indicates a neurological problem, and treatment is needed before starting or resuming an intensive training program.

The Weight-Training Readiness Form on page 15 is designed for use with both males and females. Male-only and female-only forms are available on the DVD.

There are seven parameters of a weight-training dysfunction:

1. The location of the dysfunction

There are two methods for describing the dysfunctional area: a checklist of various regions and muscles and a pain diagram that can be marked to indicate the location of pain or other signs of dysfunction such as numbness or tingling.

2. The type of pain or sensation experienced

The person can describe the pain or sensation in common terms. Four common types of sensation accompany a dysfunction: pain, tingling, numbness, and stiffness. Many more terms are used to describe pain, but these four are most used clinically.

Pain can occur in a muscle or joint. The person should point with one finger to the painful or problematic area. Pain near the joint line may indicate a problem with the joint or the muscle's tendinous attachment near the joint. A sweeping motion up and down the muscle usually indicates a muscle problem. If the person can point with exactly one finger to the area, the problem may be with a joint or a bursa. Another distinguishing factor is when the pain occurs. If pain occurs only with motion or lifting, muscles are involved. If the area is painful both at rest and in motion, it may be a bursa problem or an inflamed joint.

Tingling is an exaggerated or hypersensitive sensation originating from the nervous system. The clinical term for this is paresthesia, which is an abnormal sensation such as tingling, burning, or prickling. There are many causes for this type of sensation, which require a detailed examination to differentiate.

Numbness is the loss of sensation as a result of nerve compression or tension. A detailed examination is needed to identify the cause of the numbness.

Stiffness is the restriction of motion with a feeling of soreness, tension, or tightness. Either postworkout soreness or an alteration of the soft tissues can cause the restriction of motion.

3. The exercise, if any, that caused the dysfunction

The type of exercise that caused the dysfunction is very important. If the dysfunction occurred during a compound exercise such as a squat or a bench press, usually a number of different muscles or joints, and possibly their nerve supply, have been affected and must be rehabilitated or treated. If the dysfunction occurred during a single-joint or isolation exercise such as a leg extension or a lateral dumbbell raise, usually a single muscle is affected, with possible joint involvement. Knowing the type of exercise during which the dysfunction occurred also gives information about which joints and muscles are affected and enables appropriate rehabilitation or treatment to be performed.

4. The duration of the dysfunction

The duration of the dysfunction dramatically affects the type and duration of rehabilitation or treatment. If the dysfunction occurred within days, the main treatment focus is to reduce inflammation and prevent muscle spasms. If the dysfunction occurred within weeks, inflammation is already reduced, but an altered muscle pattern along with some scar tissue have formed. After months, no inflammation remains, but the scar tissue has altered the movement pattern of the muscle and joint. Nerves may also be involved. After years, there is no inflammation, but the altered movement pattern may have created a compensatory effect, causing other muscles to become dysfunctional. It is now harder to identify the original dysfunctional muscle.

5. The types of treatment that have worked and not worked

This information can save a lot of time, because it allows treatments that have already been used to be removed from consideration. This information can be misleading, however, because the treatment may not have been done correctly or at the right time or in combination with other necessary treatments. Just because a certain treatment was tried before does not mean that it will not work. It may need other supplemental treatments to be effective. Most injuries are multifactorial (caused by many things), so it is logical that many simultaneous types of treatment may be needed.

6. The exercises that cause pain

This question reveals what the problematic exercises have in common. It may not be apparent at first, but the response can distinguish between a muscle dysfunction and a joint dysfunction. In a muscle dysfunction, any exercise that stresses that muscle through one plane of motion will cause pain. In a joint dysfunction, any exercise that stresses that joint through various planes of motion will cause pain. For example, if a person has pain in the shoulder when bench pressing but not overhead shoulder pressing, the rotator cuff muscles may not be functioning optimally, and the pectoral muscle may also be dysfunctional. If there is pain during both bench pressing and overhead shoulder pressing, there might be a joint dysfunction that may need rehabilitation or treatment. If the primary problem is joint dysfunction, then you usually have a secondary problem of muscle dysfunction.

7. The motion and direction of motion that is painful

This question is rarely asked but is one of the most important to determine which muscle is involved and with what type of contraction. Three types of contractions occur during a lift. The muscle shortens with a concentric contraction. During an eccentric contraction, the muscle contracts while lengthening. An isometric contraction is a contraction of the muscle with no movement that occurs at the top and bottom of the exercise.

Once the direction that causes pain is known, it can be determined if the muscle is dysfunctional, if the joint is unstable, or if the nerve supply is not functioning optimally. Pain with the concentric contraction of a muscle can indicate a dysfunction with the muscle or tendon. Pain on the eccentric contraction may indicate a shortened dysfunctional muscle that is stressed. Pain during the isometric phase usually shows joint instability and a dysfunction with the nervous system in the joint and muscle.

Stress Level Questionnaire

The Subjective Training Stress Level Questionnaire determines whether training stress levels are high enough to adversely affect the adrenal glands and cause relative adrenal insufficiency symptoms. The main symptoms are being tired all the time, dull pains that do not go away, getting dizzy when going from lying to standing quickly, and sensitivity to sunlight. Any of these symptoms indicate a possible biochemical dysfunction caused by a vitamin or mineral deficiency.

Weight-Training Readiness Form

Name: _____   Date: _____

Area of Injury

❑ Neck	❑ Upper back	❑ Lower back	❑ Hip	❑ Knee	❑ Ankle
❑ Foot	❑ Shoulder	❑ Elbow	❑ Wrist	❑ Hand	❑ Chest
❑ Gluteus	❑ Quadriceps	❑ Hamstring	❑ Calf	❑ Forearm	❑ Biceps
❑ Triceps	❑ Abdomen				

Pain Diagram

Please indicate all areas of·

Pain	XXXX
Tingling	/ / / /
Numbness	OOOO
Stiffness	+ + + +

Did the injury occur on an exercise: ❑ Yes   ❑ No   ❑ Don't know

    If yes, which exercise caused the injury? ___ _____

How long have you had this injury: _____ Days _____ Weeks ____ Months _____ Years

What type of treatment has worked? _____

_____

What treatment has not worked? _____

_____

List exercises that cause pain.   Which motions are painful?

1. _____   ❑ Going up   ❑ Going down

2. _____   ❑ Going up   ❑ Going down

3. _____   ❑ Going up   ❑ Going down

Subjective Training Stress Level Questionnaire

The following questionnaire assesses whether chronic stress or overtraining is creating a condition called relative adrenal insufficiency, and causing symptoms of tiredness, weakness, and pain.

Please circle the number that best describes the intensity of symptoms.

0 = None   1 = Mild   2 = Moderate   3 = Severe

1. Decreased appetite		0 1 2 3
2. Disturbed sleep		0 1 2 3
3. Decreased strength		0 1 2 3
4. Decreased recovery following exercise		0 1 2 3
5. Increased irritability		0 1 2 3
6. When lifting, weights feel heavy		0 1 2 3
7. Increased incidence of injuries		0 1 2 3
8. Decreased immunity (e.g., catching colds easily)		0 1 2 3
9. Dizziness upon rising		0 1 2 3
10. Depression or rapid mood swings		0 1 2 3
11. Constant muscle soreness		0 1 2 3
12. Increased sensitivity to sunlight (require sunglasses)		0 1 2 3

Total _____

Training Stress Level Index

0   3   6   9   12   15   18   21   24   27   30   33   36
Mild   **Moderate**   **Severe**
                                                            (overstress)

Each answer has a number to quantify the severity of the dysfunction. These numbers are added up, and the total circled on the scoring scale. The total score determines what action is needed.

For symptoms in the mild to moderate range, rest should be increased, possibly by taking a week off from training. This helps the person recuperate and be able to train harder when training is resumed. For symptoms in the moderate to severe range, you may have a vitamin or mineral deficiency. If a doctor understands and is able treat overstress symptoms naturally with diet, vitamins, minerals, and herbs, the appropriate natural remedies are often sufficient to resolve the problem without any medication. Taking a week or two off training is also needed to recover properly.

Summary

This chapter explored the different characteristics of weight-training dysfunction and how it affects the body and training. Although weight-training technique and program design is important, determining the state of the body and its ability to handle different weight-training exercises is also important to establish. To learn this information, let's turn to the next chapter and review the assessments presented on the DVD, their scoring systems, and the rationale behind them.

2

Assessing Weight-Training Readiness

One of the main purposes of this book is to provide tests to determine a person's ability to do specific weight-training exercises. The Weight-Training Readiness Exam described here can determine whether the joints, muscles, and nerves are healthy and able to function optimally or whether there are hidden problems that may show up only in specific ranges of motion or when a load is applied to a specific area.

The Weight-Training Readiness Exam comprises of three tests: a self-test, an exercise test, and a functional muscle test. The self-test is a test that the person can do on his or her own to analyze range of motion. The exercise test involves performing specific weight-training exercises and helps determine whether any pain occurs during training and its severity. The functional muscle test is conducted by a doctor, therapist, or trainer to determine whether specific muscles are functioning optimally. Each of the three tests gives a different view of the body so that a safe and effective weight-training program can be developed.

Self-Test

The self-test can be performed at home or in a gym or fitness center. No special equipment other than eyes and a mirror is needed. Two main criteria are tested: whether range of motion is full or decreased for each weight-training exercise and whether or not the specific range of motion for each exercise causes pain.

The self-test checks for pain or decreased range of motion during exercises without weight. If an exercise's range of motion causes pain without weight, there is a good chance that it will cause even more pain with weight. When the exercise range of motion is decreased, the body may compensate by using other muscles, which can create further dysfunction in the joints by strengthening stronger, larger muscles at the expense of smaller muscles.

This test is only a guideline to find out whether limited range of motion may eventually require attention.

Scoring

A negative result—the absence of any problems—is scored as a 0, and a positive result—pain or decreased range of motion—is scored as 1. That is, normal range of motion scores 0; decreased range of motion scores 1. No pain scores 0; pain scores 1. Use the Self-Test Scoring Sheet to record the scores for each test. A sample of the Self-Test Scoring Sheet for the shoulder tests is shown here; scoring sheets for all body parts can be printed from the DVD.

For printable Self-Test Scoring Sheets for all body areas, access the forms on the DVD.

After the person has performed all the different self-tests, the answers are added to get the total score for the self-test. This clarifies whether the person is cleared for training, needs flexibility exercises, rehabilitation, or treatment to improve function. Table 2.1 provides an example of a completed Self-Test Scoring Sheet for the shoulder.

Table 2.1 Sample Shoulder Self-Test

Shoulder self-test	Test results			Functional score
	Decreased range of motion	No	Yes	
	Pain	No	Yes	
1. Dumbbell lateral raise test		0	1	2
		0	1	
2. Dumbbell shoulder press test		0	1	0
		0	1	
3. Barbell shoulder press test		0	1	0
		0	1	
4. Bent-over lateral raise test		0	1	0
		0	1	
5. Hand to opposite shoulder test		0	1	1
		0	1	
6. Hand to back of neck test		0	1	1
		0	1	
7. Hand behind the back test		0	1	1
		0	1	
8. Internal rotation test		0	1	0
		0	1	
9. External rotation test		0	1	1
		0	1	
10. Pencil test		0	1	0
		0	1	

Self-Test Scoring Sheet—Shoulder

Shoulder self-test	Test results			Functional score
	Decreased range of motion	**No**	**Yes**	
	Pain	**No**	**Yes**	
1. Dumbbell lateral raise test		0	1	
		0	1	
2. Dumbbell shoulder press test		0	1	
		0	1	
3. Barbell shoulder press test		0	1	
		0	1	
4. Bent-over lateral raise test		0	1	
		0	1	
5. Hand to opposite shoulder test		0	1	
		0	1	
6. Hand to back of neck test		0	1	
		0	1	
7. Hand behind the back test		0	1	
		0	1	
8. Internal rotation test		0	1	
		0	1	
9. External rotation test		0	1	
		0	1	
10. Pencil test		0	1	
		0	1	

Low score 1–7	Medium score 8–14	High score 15–20
Specific flexibility exercises recommended	Specific flexibility and rehabilitative exercises recommended	Treatment recommended

Self-Test Total Score

The total score indicates the severity of the dysfunction. The higher the score, the more severe the dysfunction and the harder the person will have to work to address that dysfunction. If the score is low, function can usually be improved through flexibility exercises. A medium score indicates a need for some flexibility work along with some rehabilitative exercises to help strengthen the affected muscles. A high score means that the person needs treatment because he or she has a fair amount of pain and decreased range of motion throughout different exercises. This score gives an idea of a person's functional status; it is not intended as a diagnosis of any disease or injury. For a score of 2 on any test, the exercise test is recommended to determine the functional level.

Table 2.2 shows how to score the self-test. If the total score is 6, for example, put a 6 in the self-test total score box, which indicates that flexibility exercises are recommended for those positive tests.

Table 2.2   Sample Shoulder Self-Test Results

Total score	Low score 0-7	Medium score 8-14	High score 15-20
6	Specific flexibility exercises recommended	Specific flexibility and rehabilitative exercises recommended	Treatment recommended

Exercise Test

During the exercise test, the person does actual weight-training exercises to determine whether there is any pain associated with the exercise, and how the pain affects training. The exercise test also determines the level of function.

If the person experiences any pain during the exercise, it is important to first ensure that he or she uses the proper exercise technique. In many cases, improper exercise technique, not the muscle or joint itself, causes pain.

Functional Scoring System

The functional scoring system indicates the level of functioning and pain and how it affects training. The four different levels are as follows:

- Functional level 0 (FL0): No pain during the exercise.
- Functional level 1 (FL1): The joint and muscles in the body part being used feel tight, but the muscle feels better at the end of the workout. The tightness does not affect the weight lifted.
- Functional level 2 (FL2): Pain is increased when training and remains after the workout. It necessitates the use of a lighter weight in this exercise.
- Functional level 3 (FL3): Severe pain completely prevents performance of the exercise. Because movement is too painful, the exercise must be cut from the weight-training routine.

Table 2.3 demonstrates how to determine the functional level of the shoulder. If the person scores 2 on the self-test, one set of 10 repetitions of the same exercise as in the self-test should be done. If the shoulder feels strong and painfree at the beginning and end of the set, the score is FL0. If the shoulder feels tight at the beginning of the set and better at the end of the set, the score is FL1, and flexibility exercises specific to that motion are indicated. If the shoulder feels worse at the end of the set, the score is FL2, and flexibility and rehabilitation exercises specific to that motion are indicated. If the person cannot even do the exercise because of pain, the score is FL3, and appropriate treatment for the painful area should be sought.

Table 2.3   Sample Exercise Test Scoring Sheet

Shoulder exercise test	Funtional Level			
1. Dumbbell lateral raise test	FL0	FL1	(FL2)	FL3
2. Dumbbell shoulder press test	FL0	(FL1)	FL2	FL3
3. Barbell shoulder press test	FL0	(FL1)	FL2	FL3
4. Bent-over lateral raise test	(FL0)	FL1	FL2	FL3

Use the following sample Exercise Test Scoring Sheet to record the scores for each shoulder test by circling the applicable level. Scoring sheets for each body part can be printed from the DVD.

For printable Exercise Test Scoring Sheets for all body areas, access the forms on the DVD.

Improving the Functional Level

Once the functional level has been determined, if it is not optimal, improvements need to be made through exercise modification, flexibility exercises, rehabilitative exercises, or treatment. It is most important to check weight-training technique. Someone with a good working knowledge of weight-training exercises may be needed to watch the person to determine if poor technique is the cause of pain. The observer should have a fairly high level of understanding of weight training. Just because someone weight-trains does not mean he or she knows how to do it properly. Sometimes poor advice is worse than no advice. The observer should be well qualified, either through certification courses, competition at a high level, or many years of experience helping others.

Functional Level 0
Functional level 0 indicates optimal range of motion and function with no pain and the person is cleared to do the weight-training exercise.

Functional Level 1
Functional level 1 indicates that the joint and muscles feel tight when training, usually due to tightness or possible shortening of the muscle. This type of tightness can usually be remedied through flexibility exercises for various muscles in

Exercise Test Scoring Sheet—Shoulder

Shoulder exercise test	Functional Level			
1. Dumbbell lateral raise test	FL0	FL1	FL2	FL3
2. Dumbbell shoulder press test	FL0	FL1	FL2	FL3
3. Barbell shoulder press test	FL0	FL1	FL2	FL3
4. Bent-over lateral raise test	FL0	FL1	FL2	FL3

FL0	No pain during the exercise. Continue training.
FL1	The joint and muscles in the body part being trained feel tight, but the muscle feels better at the end of the workout. The tightness does not affect the weight lifted. Specific flexibility exercise recommended.
FL2	Pain is increased when training and remains after the workout. It necessitates the use of a lighter weight in this exercise. Specific flexibility and rehabilitation exercise recommended.
FL3	Severe pain completely prevents performance of the exercise. Because the movement is too painful, the exercise must be cut from the weight-training routine. Treatment recommended.

the body part. The flexibility exercises recommended to improve performance of specific weight-training exercises are demonstrated on the DVD. These stretches can be incorporated into the daily stretching routine.

Functional Level 2
Functional level 2 indicates that increasing pain is experienced during the weight-training exercise. The dysfunction clearly goes beyond just tight muscles in this case. Certain muscles are not only tight but have become damaged and weakened. This is why a lighter weight is needed for the exercise. The solution is flexibility and rehabilitation exercises.

Functional Level 3
Functional level 3 indicates that severe pain is causing a complete inability to perform the exercise. The movement is too painful, usually due to a muscle, joint, and nerve problem or a combination of them. An assessment for treatment is warranted. Some flexibility and rehabilitation exercises can be attempted and the problematic weight-training exercise avoided, but proper treatment of the muscle, joint, and nerve can accelerate improvement in function.

Exercises to Improve Functional Level
Exercise technique modification allows the person to continue to do a form of the exercise that causes less stress. The modification can be a change in the angle of the arm, position of the hand, range of motion, foot stance width, or the angle to which the back is bent. These changes allow the person to continue to do the exercise while rehabilitating and stretching the affected area until the person can once again do the exercise in the original style. In some instances the exercise must be dropped altogether during rehabilitation and strengthening. Exercise technique modifications are discussed in chapter 4.

Rehabilitation exercises are needed if the muscle has been traumatized or damaged to the point that it is difficult to contract properly. When certain smaller muscles become damaged, the larger prime mover muscles take over and create muscle imbalances. If muscle or joint dysfunction causes muscle imbalances, the weight-training exercise movement may become unstable at certain points, thereby increasing the risk of injury and pain. To exercise the small supporting muscles, specific exercise positions and movements allow those muscles to fire instead of the prime movers. Because the extent of muscle weakness or damage is not known, it is best to start with the lowest amount of tension on the muscle, then slowly increase it.

Three different levels of rehabilitative exercises can strengthen the muscle and potentially improve function: isometric agonist-antagonist contractions, active proprioceptive neuromuscular facilitation (PNF), and resistive tubing exercises. Isometric agonist-antagonist exercises are static contractions of the muscle that involve no motion and exercise opposite muscle groups. Active PNF involves a range of motion with resistance forward and backward in an X pattern across the body. Resistive tubing exercises are performed with a piece of rubber tubing that is anchored at one end and has a handle at the other end to perform the same exercise range of motion that is causing the pain or weakness. A more detailed description of these exercises is provided in chapter 5 and demonstrated on the DVD.

Functional Muscle Test

Functional muscle testing evaluates how well the muscles in the body are functioning. Many books have been written about functional muscle testing from different perspectives. The type of functional muscle test discussed here determines how well the muscles function that are used in the exercise plane of motion. In any weight-training exercise, many muscles contract all at the same time in various degrees, depending on the range of motion. Throughout each repetition, specific muscles contract maximally at different times and then decrease contraction to make the movement smooth and continuous. Research has shown that muscle contraction patterns change throughout a weight-training set also due to fatigue. This is important for treating complicated weight-training injuries.

Functional muscle testing that is administered by a doctor, therapist, or trainer can reveal further dysfunctions in the muscle, joint, or nerve complex. Functional muscle testing helps to determine which of three possible causes for muscle weakness are present:

1. The muscle may be deconditioned or damaged to the point that it has adhesions, is maladaptively shortened, is neurologically inhibited by an antagonist muscle, or has become deconditioned.

2. The joint has an altered range of motion or position, causing the muscles that cross that joint to be inhibited neurologically causing a potential muscle weakness.

3. The nerve is compressed or under abnormal tension. Any abnormal vertebral motion or position can decrease the potential of neurological impulses from the spine to the extremities and thus decrease the ability to contract the muscles properly. The chiropractic term for this condition is vertebral subluxation. Nerve entrapment syndrome occurs when a nerve is either compressed or overstretched from hypertonic muscles as it goes down the arm or leg.

Functional muscle testing assesses the neurological system. The normal response to the functional muscle test is normal facilitation or normal inhibition. The muscle turns on and contracts, (is facilitated) and off with no contraction (is inhibited) properly and at the right time under neurological control. An abnormal response to the functional muscle test might be abnormal facilitation, in which the muscle is overfacilitated and contracts too much and spasms. Another abnormal response is abnormal inhibition, in which the muscles stay in an inhibited state and do not contract to their full potential. The terms *weak* and *strong* are commonly used instead of normal *inhibition* and *facilitation* in muscle testing, so the terms *weak* and *strong* are used in this book and on the DVD for simplicity. However, *weak* and *strong* should not be confused with meanings related to conditioning; in this context they refer to the neurological system's functional ability to adapt to an increased force temporarily.

The amount of force or strength the tester applies during this test depends on several factors. One is the size of the person and muscle being tested. Another is whether the person being tested is physically fit and strong or physically unfit and weak. This is not a test of strength but a test to see whether the neuromuscular system can adapt to an increased force (i.e., the ability of the muscle to maintain resistance against the tester without moving the limb). If the muscle is able to maintain resistance in the correct test position, this is considered a strong muscle or a normal response. If the muscle is unable to maintain its normal force and maintain the correct test position, this is a weak muscle or abnormal response.

The person tested is positioned so that only one muscle or muscle group is primarily being tested with decreased support from other synergistic muscle groups. The tester must use his or her judgment and kinesthetic feedback from the person to avoid applying too much force and getting a false positive response.

Scoring

Functional muscle testing can determine whether a muscle is weak and experiences pain when tested. A muscle may be weak with no pain, or a strong muscle may have pain. One does not imply the other. Any weak and painful muscle is usually a red flag that the area needs to be assessed further to determine if treatment is warranted. These functional test scores are only guidelines to give an idea of what is occurring inside the body. Table 2.4 demonstrates how to use the Functional Test Scoring Sheets.

Table 2.4   Sample Functional Muscle Test Scoring Sheet

Shoulder functional muscle test	Test results		Functional muscle test score
	Strong	Weak	
Serratus anterior	(0)	1	0
Lateral deltoid	0	(1)	1
Anterior deltoid	(0)	1	0
Posterior deltoid	(0)	1	0
Infraspinatus	0	(1)	1
Subscapularis	(0)	1	0
Teres minor	(0)	1	0
Supraspinatus	(0)	1	0
Subclavius	(0)	1	0

Low score—1 One muscle weak	Medium score—2 Two muscles weak	High score—3 Three or more muscles weak
Muscle dysfunction; flexibility exercises recommended	Muscle/joint dysfunction; flexibility and rehabilitative exercises recommended	Muscle/joint/nerve dysfunction; flexibility and rehabilitative exercises and possible treatment recommended

Functional Muscle Test Scoring Sheet—Shoulder

Shoulder functional muscle test	Test results		Functional muscle test score
	Strong	Weak	
Serratus anterior	0	1	
Lateral deltoid	0	1	
Anterior deltoid	0	1	
Posterior deltoid	0	1	
Infraspinatus	0	1	
Subscapularis	0	1	
Teres minor	0	1	
Supraspinatus	0	1	
Subclavius	0	1	

Low score—1 One muscle weak	Medium score—2 Two muscles weak	High score—3 Three or more muscles weak
Muscle dysfunction; flexibility exercises recommended	Muscle/joint dysfunction; flexibility and rehabilitative exercises recommended	Muscle/joint/nerve dysfunction; flexibility and rehabilitative exercises and possible treatment recommended

A low test score generally means that only one muscle is weak and possibly only a muscle dysfunction needs to be addressed. A medium test score indicates that two muscles are weak in a joint complex and both a muscle and joint dysfunction may be present. A high score indicates that three or more muscles in the joint complex are weak and there is a muscle, joint, and nerve dysfunction present, therefore just one type of treatment or exercise will not be able to address them all.

For printable Functional Muscle Test Scoring Sheets for each body area, access the forms on the DVD.

Use the sample Functional Muscle Test Scoring Sheet to record the scores for each test. Scoring sheets for each body part can be printed from the DVD.

How the Functional Muscle Test Works

It is important to use the proper amount of force during functional muscle testing to determine muscle function. Figure 2.1 shows an example of testing a lateral deltoid muscle; the solid line shows the force applied by the tester, and the dashed line shows the resisting force from the person being tested. The person being tested assumes the muscle testing position by extending the arm horizontally and holding it in this abducted position with an upward force. The tester resists this upward force by pushing down with his or her hand on the arm with the same amount of force. The arm does not move because both forces are the same; this phase of the muscle test lasts about one or two seconds. In the second phase of the test, the tester increases the downward force by approximately five pounds to see if the muscle being tested can adapt to the slight increase of force. If the muscle adapts neurologically to the increased force, it has no functional weaknesses; this is a normal muscle test result (figure 2.1a). If the person cannot adapt neurologically to the extra five pounds of force, then this is an abnormal test result (figure 2.1b) with functional weaknesses. The muscle cannot adapt to the extra force and moves or "breaks" the horizontal isometric arm position and the arm moves downward towards the floor.

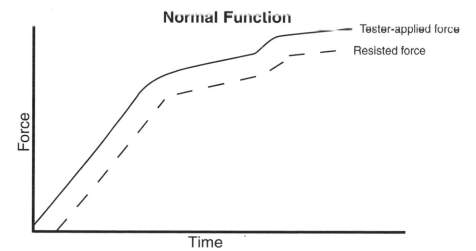

Figure 2.1a Normal functional muscle test result.

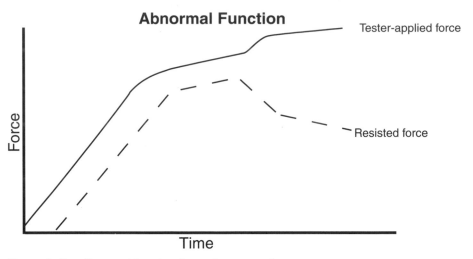

Figure 2.1b Abnormal functional muscle test result.

Treatment of Weight-Training Dysfunctions

When it has been determined that you have a weight-training dysfunction, many different types of treatment providers are available: medical doctors, chiropractors, physical therapists, osteopaths, massage therapists, athletic trainers, and so on. Most professions use different types of treatments. Instead of deciding what type of provider to see, it is better to determine the type of treatment that would be most beneficial, although the treatment is only as good as the person delivering it. Get referrals from people who have received excellent treatment and referrals from other health professionals as to who are the best with specific treatment techniques and protocols for weight-training dysfunctions. A professional with a good understanding of the mechanics of weight training and how it can affect muscle function may diagnose problems more accurately. Remember, the treatment is usually only as good as the person delivering it.

Chapter 1 discussed the four main types of weight-training dysfunctions: muscle, joint, nerve, and biochemical. Since every dysfunction is unique, the list below offers a general description and guidance and should not be taken as an absolute prescription for the various types of treatment and how effective they are for these dysfunctions.

- **Massage therapy** is the manipulation of the soft tissues of the body to optimize those tissues by increasing blood circulation, reducing muscle tension, and improving circulation of blood and lymph movement. It consists of different hands-on manual techniques that include applying fixed or movable pressure to the body. This treatment is very beneficial for muscle dysfunctions.

- **Myofascial therapy** decreases the tension in the fibrous bands of connective tissue, or fascia, that encase muscles throughout the body. Injury or adhesions to this network of fascia can be a major cause of pain and impeded motion. In myofascial therapy the fascia is loaded with a constant force in a specific direction until a release occurs, aiming to alleviate these problems by breaking up constrictions in the fascia. This therapy is very beneficial for muscle dysfunctions.

■ **Active release technique (ART)** is a soft-tissue system that treats problems with the muscles, tendons, ligaments, fascia, and nerves. These problems often result from overuse injuries, causing an accumulation of small tears (microtrauma) to produce abnormal dense scar tissue in the affected area. The abnormal tissues are treated by combining a precisely directed tension with very specific body movements to free restricted tissues and reduce the amount of scar tissue. This therapy is very beneficial for muscle and joint dysfunctions and nerve entrapments.

■ **Percussion therapy** is a steady application of a rhythmic mechanical force with an instrument to induce a harmonic vibration in the restricted fascial tissues until they release. This treatment is very beneficial for muscle dysfunctions.

■ **Chiropractic adjustment** is a very specific and precisely executed manual force directed at a dysfunctional spinal joint or subluxation (an abnormal functional or structural joint complex that compromises neural integrity), with the objective to restore normal joint and nerve function. The spinal joints are richly innervated by nerves, which have direct connections to the spinal cord and major nerve pathways supplying every tissue and organ in the body. A subluxation can have considerable impact on one's health. Chiropractic adjustments are very beneficial for joint and nerve dysfunctions.

■ **Microcurrent therapy** is an instrument that uses the same electrical current (microamps—millionths of an amp) as your own cells to increase its own energy ATP production (increases up to 500%), increasing protein synthesis and waste product removal. Different microcurrent frequencies can be used to decrease the scar tissue and dysfunction of the muscle tissue. This therapy is very beneficial for muscle dysfunctions.

■ **Electronic muscle stimulation (EMS)** is an instrument that uses different electrical current parameters (frequency, intensity, and waveform) to increase strength in injured muscles by stimulating motor nerves to initiate and hold muscles in a contracted state. It is useful in injury cases involving immobilization of a joint or contraindication to dynamic exercise. EMS is very beneficial for muscle and nerve dysfunctions.

■ **Acupuncture** is the insertion of very fine needles into the skin to stimulate specific points called acupuncture points. These points can stimulate the nervous system to decrease muscle spasms and also release narcotic-like substances called endorphins, which reduce pain. Acupuncture is very beneficial for muscle and nerve dysfunctions.

■ **Cold laser therapy** is laser-light energy that penetrates the skin and is absorbed by micromolecules in the body. The light energy photons are then transformed into biochemical energy and initiate a cascade of events at a cellular level to restore normal cellular function called biomodulation. Biomodulation is the stimulation of cells and tissues to bring them to their most natural state. The laser also increases ATP production, reduces pain by endorphin release, and increases collagen formation for faster wound healing. This therapy is very beneficial for muscle and nerve dysfunctions.

- **Ultrasound therapy** is an instrument that penetrates the body by using ultrasound energy from the acoustic or sound spectrum (undetectable to the human ear). This type of therapy produces heat for pain relief and stimulates repair to muscle tissue and other connective tissue such as ligaments and tendons. Ultrasound therapy is very beneficial for muscle and joint dysfunctions.

- **Dietary supplements** are essential nutrients for optimal performance of strength and muscular development. These are nutrients such as vitamins, minerals, herbs, proteins and amino acids, essential fatty acids, and other similar nutritional substances that are very beneficial for biochemical dysfunctions.

- **Drugs or medications** are any natural or artificially made chemical that are used to treat, prevent, or alleviate the symptoms of inflammation and disease. These are very beneficial for biochemical dysfunctions.

Summary

This chapter discussed the Weight-Training Readiness Exam, which includes three different types of tests. These tests will help determine the body's functional level and how it may affect training. The assessment scores can be used to design a training program to improve function through either flexibility or rehabilitation exercises or appropriate treatment. Next, we will look at functional anatomy. This chapter will review where the muscles used in training are located, how they function, and how specific muscle weaknesses are manifested in the body. The next chapter also links muscles to exercise movement and discusses optimal training techniques for each exercise.

3

Linking Muscles to Exercise Movement

A good review of how each muscle functions, independently and together with other muscles, is important for developing a proper weight-training program. Functional anatomy examines where a muscle originates, where it inserts, and how it functions to move the body.

These concepts of functional anatomy can be applied to different training techniques for each muscle group for optimal muscular development and strength. Functional anatomy concepts help link the muscles to exercise movements.

For specific exercise tests and exercise techniques, see the specific body areas on the DVD.

This chapter also discusses how anatomy affects functionality and how weaknesses manifest in the body if the muscle or joint structure does not function optimally. For example, when the biceps muscle contracts to flex the elbow, the synergistic muscles that help with elbow flexion are the brachialis and brachioradialis. For the biceps muscle to fully contract, the antagonistic muscle that needs to relax is the triceps muscle. When all these muscle work together properly, the movement is powerful, smooth, and precise. If any of the muscles are not functioning properly, then the movement becomes weak, unstable, and imprecise. If the triceps does not relax but stays contracted and hypertonic, elbow flexion is decreased and may even cause pain. This type of anatomical information can be used to detect reduced functionality and may give clues about what to look for if an exercise is difficult to perform.

Deltoid Muscle

The deltoid is a muscle with three different heads: anterior, lateral, and posterior. The anterior deltoid arises from the lateral third of the clavicle and inserts into the deltoid tubercle of the humerus. Its main action is humeral flexion, and it cooperates with the pectoralis major in drawing the arm forward.

The lateral deltoid arises from the acromion process and inserts into deltoid tubercle of the humerus. Its main action is abduction of the humerus. It is the strongest of the three heads and is aided by the supraspinatus in abduction and limited by the tightening of the lower shoulder capsule. As the arm is abducted, the lateral deltoid contracts, while the anterior and posterior deltoid are stretched, steadying the limb and preventing any sideways motion.

The posterior deltoid arises from the lateral aspect of the spine of the scapula and inserts into the deltoid tubercle of the humerus. Its main action is humeral extension, and it assists the latissimus dorsi and teres major in drawing the arm backward into extension.

Indications of Weakness

If the anterior deltoid is weakened, overhead presses become difficult and painful. A weakness can occur also if there is an acromioclavicular (AC) joint sprain since the anterior deltoid muscle cannot contract properly in an unstable joint.

If range of motion in abduction is decreased, the infraspinatus and pectoralis major may have shortened and may not allow full motion of the arm. Fixation of the scapula to the thoracic wall can also decrease the amount of arm abduction. Sprain of the AC joint can weaken the lateral deltoid muscle since muscles cannot contract properly in an unstable joint.

The posterior deltoid is weakened when the anterior deltoid and pectoralis muscles become shortened and hypertonic, causing agonist–antagonist muscle inhibition. If the glenohumeral joint has shifted forward due to the shortened muscles, it needs to be either treated or stretched to allow the posterior deltoid to contract properly again.

Optimal Training Principles

The shoulder joint is unique in that it relies on muscles and ligaments instead of the skeletal system for its stability. This allows for a large range of motion in the joint, but also makes it more susceptible to injury. Therefore, it is very important to develop all the muscles in the shoulder region to prevent injuries.

To fully develop the entire deltoid muscle with emphasis on the lateral head, the barbell or dumbbell shoulder press with the elbows out to the side is excellent for those with optimal shoulder range of motion. The anterior deltoid is trained frequently because of its involvement in chest work. Exercises specifically for anterior deltoid, such as front raises, are usually not needed except for rehabilitation or specific strength training purposes.

The dumbbell lateral raise is an excellent isolation exercise that can be further enhanced by customizing it for each person's biomechanics and muscle insertions. The lateral head in many people is more posterior than directly lateral. In that case, bending forward slightly optimally positions the lateral deltoid for exercise. The technique of turning the thumb down at the top of the lateral dumbbell raise also activates more lateral fibers, but it may be safer to change the body position. The thumb-down lateral raise can potentially create an impingement in the AC joint in the shoulder.

To take pressure off the lower back when performing a posterior deltoid raise, the person can sit on the end of a bench with the dumbbells under the thighs and then bring the dumbbells out laterally until the arms are parallel to the floor.

Training with barbells and dumbbells instead of machines allows the development of all the small, synergistic rotator cuff muscles that also needed strengthening. These small muscles are rarely exercised in machines since the fixed plane and range of motion offered by machines decreases the need for stabilization.

Rotator Cuff Muscles

The rotator cuff comprises of four muscles: the subscapularis, infraspinatus, teres minor, and supraspinatus.

The subscapularis muscle arises from the inner surface of the scapula and inserts on the anterior humerus at the lesser tubercle and inferior shoulder capsule. Its main action is internal rotation of the humerus, and it also assists in humerus adduction. It also stabilizes the humeral head in the glenoid cavity during arm abduction.

The infraspinatus arises from the posterior medial surface of the scapula below the spine of the scapula, and it inserts into the greater tuberosity of the humerus and the shoulder joint capsule. Its main action is to externally rotate the arm, along with the teres minor. It assists in stabilizing the head of the humerus in the glenoid cavity while the arm is elevated; the superior fibers aid in abduction, and the inferior fibers in adduction.

The teres minor arises from the axillary border of the scapula on the dorsal surface, and it inserts into the inferior aspect of the greater tuberosity of the humerus. Its main action is to externally rotate the arm, along with the infraspinatus. It assists in stabilizing the head of the humerus in the glenoid cavity while the arm is elevated.

The supraspinatus arises from the medial two-thirds of the supraspinatus fossa on the scapula and inserts into the greater tubercle of the humerus. Its main function is to assist in abducting the humerus and to hold the head of the humerus in the glenoid fossa.

Indications of Weakness

Weakness of the infraspinatus muscle may cause shortening and hypertonicity of the subscapularis muscle due to agonist–antagonistic interaction (the amount of contraction by the agonist is partially dictated by how much the antagonist can relax). This problem can be identified by the scapula's seeming to pull laterally when the arm is abducted. This is caused by the shortened subscapularis muscle.

Shortening and hypertonicity of the subscapularis decreases range of motion of the humerus and, if severe enough, can manifest as a frozen shoulder or adhesive capsulitis. The subscapularis muscle often gets many adhesions from excessive bench-pressing, which may be felt as pain in the front of the shoulder. This pain is caused by the subscapularis muscle's preventing the head of the humerus from moving forward when the bench-press bar is at the chest. This puts undue stress on the subscapularis, which often becomes inflamed. Inflammation creates adhesions and scar tissue, weakening the muscle.

Weakness of the teres minor muscle may cause internal rotation of the arm when relaxed at the side while the person is standing. A shortened or hypertonic teres minor decreases the ability to reach behind the back.

Weakness of the supraspinatus muscle can cause difficulty raising and keeping the arm parallel to the floor. If the muscle is extremely weak, the torso bends laterally to initiate abduction of the arm. Shoulder joint crepitus, or noise in the joint, is often due to adhesions in this muscle. This muscle has a poor blood supply and is often damaged at the myotendinous junction, causing shoulder pain and weakness.

Optimal Training Principles

When working the rotator cuff muscles, it is important to identify muscles that are weak and underdeveloped and ones that are shortened and overdeveloped. In general, if there is an imbalance, the subscapularis muscle is shortened and overdeveloped and the infraspinatus and teres minor muscles are underdeveloped and weak.

One of the most common causes of a supraspinatus injury is a dysfunctional subscapularis muscle. The subscapularis muscle holds the head of the humerus posteriorly and inferiorly during pushing movements such as the bench press. When the subscapularis becomes dysfunctional, it allows the head of the humerus to move anteriorly and superiorly, thus causing injury and weakness to the supraspinatus via impingement on the acromion.

The infraspinatus exercise, described on the DVD, is best performed with a pulley system since there will be tension at the bottom and top of the exercise. The second best would be tubing since it has little tension at the bottom, but maximum tension at the top. The dumbbell version is the most popular, but least preferred since there is maximum tension on the bottom of the exercise and decreases substantially once the arm approaches perpendicular and gravity takes over. The tension is now vertical instead of horizontal, thus decreasing the amount of stress on the infraspinatus muscle.

The subscapularis exercise is best performed with a pulley system rather than tubing or dumbbells since there will be tension at the bottom and top of the exercise. An advanced version of the exercise, the cable comes from the front at a 45-degree angle, and the humerus internally rotates until the palm faces downward; then the person brings the whole arm backward until it is behind the body. This works the subscapularis through a full range of motion.

The teres minor exercise, described on the DVD, works well with a pulley system or tubing, or it can be done with a dumbbell while the person lies on one side and externally rotates the humerus.

The supraspinatus exercise can be performed with either a pulley system, tubing, or weights as they are all equally effective. The person positions the arm at a 45-

degree angle from the side of the body and then raises the arm until it is shoulder height. Whether to do the exercise with the thumb up or down for maximum isolation of the supraspinatus is controversial. Yoshitsugu and others (2002) did EMG research to explore whether internal or external rotation of the arm made a difference for isolating the supraspinatus. Their results revealed that it makes no difference and that the thumb-up position (external rotation) carries less risk of shoulder impingement than the thumb-down position (internal rotation).

All rotator cuff exercises should be done at the end of the workout or on an off day. This prevents fatigue of the small stabilizing rotator cuff muscles, which are needed when using the larger muscles, such as the pectorals or deltoids, for pressing movements.

Chest Muscles

The chest muscle group is composed of two separate muscles: the pectoralis major (clavicular and sternal head), and the pectoralis minor.

The clavicular pectoralis major arises from the anterior surface of the clavicle and inserts into the greater tubercle of the humerus and along the bicipital groove. The clavicular pectoralis major adducts the humerus horizontally across the chest and also assists in flexion of the humerus. The clavicular pectoralis major works closely with the sternal pectoralis major when the arm is extended back in a dumbbell fly position. As the arm is drawn forward, the stress shifts from the sternal fibers to the clavicular fibers until the arm is held in front.

The sternal pectoralis major arises from the lateral sternum, the cartilage of the second to the seventh ribs, and the aponeurosis of the external oblique and rectus abdominis muscles and inserts into the greater tubercle of the humerus and along the bicipital groove. The sternal pectoralis major adducts the humerus across the chest so that the arm motion is toward the opposite hip, and it also assists in flexion of the humerus. The pectoralis and anterior deltoid work closely together to flex the arm horizontally from the side to the front, as in a push-up or bench press.

The pectoralis minor arises from the third, fourth, and fifth ribs near the junction of the rib and its costal cartilage, and it inserts into the coracoid process of the scapula. It flexes the shoulder joint and draws the scapula anteriorly and inferiorly.

Indications of Weakness

If the sternal or clavicular pectoral muscles become shortened, shoulder range of motion in abduction and flexion decreases. This makes the bench press and dumbbell fly difficult and painful to do. If the clavicular pectoralis is weak, the person may experience pain around the clavicle. If the sternal pectoralis is weak, the shoulder can appear to be posterior and slightly superior from its normal position. If both pectoralis major muscles are shortened, the arm internally rotates and causes the palm to face backward instead of toward the thigh when relaxed in a standing position. If the pectoralis minor is shortened, it can cause winging of the scapula and also draw the glenohumeral joint forward, creating a biomechanical shoulder problem for weight training.

Optimal Training Principles

Start with compound movements, such as the barbell or dumbbell bench press, to strengthen and develop the pectoral muscles. To extend the elbows further back for a fuller range of motion on the bench press with less stress on the shoulder capsule, the elbows should be dropped to a 45-degree angle from the body. The dumbbell fly and pec deck focus on the pectoral muscles with decreased triceps activity.

Research has shown that even small changes in grip width (1–2 inches) in the bench press were significant in terms of muscle involvement. One of the best and safest grip widths is with the forearm perpendicular to the floor at the bottom of the lift. This grip is wide enough to stress the pectoral muscles but stress the wrist less than very wide grips do. A wide grip in the bench press increases the involvement of the sternal pectoralis and anterior deltoid. The wide grip allows the pectoral muscles to be lengthened during more of the lift and to contribute more to a successful completion of the movement. It also decreases the length of arm stroke on the ascent; the weight does not need to be lifted as far. The pectorals are most active in the bench press during the first two-thirds of the lift.

A narrow grip in the bench press takes stress off the pectorals and puts more on the triceps. When the bar is first pressed off the chest, there is a large burst of activity by the triceps along with the pectoral and anterior deltoid muscles. Then triceps activity decreases till the final one-third of the bench press to lockout.

The incline bench press decreases stress on the sternal pectoralis and puts more on the clavicular pectoralis. An incline of 30 degrees or more is needed to stress the upper chest. Arching the back should be avoided in the incline bench press. Arching tends to flatten the chest so that the larger and more powerful sternal pectoralis is used in place of the smaller clavicular pectoralis.

Depending on the amount of chest work done, it is important to train the external shoulder rotator muscles to prevent internal rotation of the arm and potential shoulder pain. Exercises to strengthen the infraspinatus and teres minor can be helpful one to two times a week at the end of the chest workout.

Different exercises and machines should be rotated in the training routine to avoid overloading the same plane and range of motion. Lack of variation can create a strength disparity among parts of the same muscle, thereby decreasing its strength and increasing risk of injury.

Biceps Muscles

The biceps muscle group is composed of two muscles: the short and long heads of the biceps and the brachialis.

The short head of the biceps arises from the tip of the coracoid process of the scapula and inserts into the radial tuberosity. The long head of the biceps arises from the supraglenoid tubercle of the scapula and inserts into the radial tuberosity. The biceps is biarticular, meaning that it crosses two joints. It is the main flexor of the elbow and has a weak flexion effect on the shoulder. The long head also helps keep the head of the humerus from rising during contraction of the deltoid. The biceps is also a strong supinator secondarily, and elbow flexion is more effective in the supinated than the pronated position.

The brachialis arises from the anterior lower half of the humerus and inserts into the ulnar tuberosity. It is uniarticular and exclusively a flexor of the elbow. Its activity is the same whether the arm is supinated or pronated since it attaches to the ulna, which does not rotate.

Indications of Weakness

A relaxed arm that hangs excessively straight or hyperextended may indicate biceps weakness. Biceps weakness may also make it difficult to supinate the forearm when the arm is moving into flexion.

If the biceps or brachialis muscle has shortened, full arm extension or supination becomes difficult, which impairs strength and muscular development. Triceps strength can also decrease if the biceps has shortened and is hypertonic because of the agonist–antagonist relationship between these two muscles.

Optimal Training Principles

Use a variety of barbell, dumbbell, and cable exercises to work various parts of the biceps. The barbell keeps the arm in a neutral position throughout the arm flexion movement, while the dumbbells and cables allow arm flexion and supination.

Three different biceps curl exercises cover different ranges of motion to fully recruit different motor units in the biceps muscle (Poliquin). The preacher curl emphasizes the first part of elbow flexion, the standing barbell curls stresses the midrange, and the concentration curl optimally stresses the last range of flexion. These three exercises increase the muscle fiber stress to not only increase the size of the muscle but also make it more functional through a full range of motion. In any biceps curl, it is important to fully extend the arm before starting the next repetition. The prestretched position of the biceps stresses the muscle through its full range of motion.

The barbell and dumbbell curls stress the brachialis and short head of the biceps at the expense of the long head of the biceps since the elbow is often in front of the body in these exercises. If the arm is behind the upper body, as in an incline dumbbell curl, the long head of the biceps is stressed more, which increases its strength and development. A functional muscle test can reveal weakness of the long head of the biceps, which is often a hidden cause of bench-press shoulder injuries. To strengthen the long head of the biceps, the person can do regular barbell or dumbbell curls to full arm flexion and then raise the elbows to shoulder height while contracting the biceps even more.

The brachialis muscle lies between the biceps and triceps and can be seen on the outer side of developed arms. The brachialis is uniarticular and exclusively a flexor of the elbow. It contracts along with the biceps whether the arm is supinated or pronated since it attaches to the ulna, which does not rotate. Because the biceps is 20 to 30 percent weaker in pronation, reverse curls with an E-Z curl bar or dumbbell hammer curls in a semipronated (thumb-up) position throughout the exercise increase the stress on the brachialis.

Biceps supination is best done just before the elbow is at 90 degrees of flexion during a dumbbell curl. If supination starts when the arm is at the side, the supinator muscle in the anterior elbow joint does most of the work, diminishing the stress on the biceps muscle.

In the book *The Body Moveable,* David Gorman states that the strength of the biceps varies with the position of the arm relative to the shoulder. For example, when the arm is above the shoulder and pulling the body up in a chin-up exercise, arm flexion strength is 83 kilograms (183 pounds). If the arm is level with the shoulder as in a horizontal preacher curl, arm flexion strength is 66 kilograms (146 pounds). If the arm is hanging down to the side, as in a barbell curl, arm flexion strength is 52 kilograms (115 pounds). Because arm flexion strength is higher with the arm above the shoulder than below, chin-ups are one of the better biceps exercises if the person is strong enough to pull up his or her body weight.

Triceps Muscle

The triceps is one muscle with three heads: the long head, the lateral head, and the medial head. The long head arises from the scapular infraglenoid tubercle. The medial head arises from medial and posterior distal humerus. The lateral head arises from the lateral and posterior proximal humerus. All three heads join to insert into the posterior surface of the ulnar olecranon.

The triceps extends the elbow, and the long head extends the arm behind the body. The medial head is active in all arm extension, while the lateral head and long head have minimal action except when the extension is forceful.

Indications of Weakness

If the triceps becomes shortened, the range of motion of elbow flexion decreases. Shortening and hypertonicity of the triceps can also decrease strength in the biceps neurologically, due to the muscles' interaction as agonist and antagonist.

Numbness, tingling, or weakness in the arm, forearm, or hand indicate possible radial nerve entrapment in the shoulder due to the shortening of the triceps long head compressing the nerve. Weakness in the triceps can cause problems with locking out the bench press or overhead shoulder press.

Optimal Training Principles

When a triceps exercise routine is set up, it is important to understand how the triceps is involved in movements with and without resistance. In triceps extension without resistance, the medial head is the workhorse and is always active, the lateral head contracts minimally, and the long head is virtually inactive. In triceps extension with resistance, the medial head is involved even more, and the lateral and long heads are recruited to aid. The lateral and long heads are reserved for heavily resisted elbow extension.

It is important to train all three triceps heads with a variety of exercises in different planes and ranges of motion. Exercising the long head, known as the lazy head, requires a lot of weight. This head fully contracts only when the weight is in the five-eight repetition range and is maximally stressed in exercises such as the close-grip bench press or the lying E-Z curl triceps extension. The lateral head is recruited more with the narrow-grip triceps push-down and the dumbbell kickback. The medial head is used in most exercises, but especially in dumbbell kickbacks and heavy overhead presses.

The researcher, Currier, discovered that the triceps isometrically contracts the most at 90 degrees of arm flexion. The exercises that best mimic that position are the close-grip bench press, dips, and triceps push-downs, which all have external torque patterns that peak at close to 90 degrees of arm flexion. The triceps kickback has a reverse torque pattern, overloads the triceps at its weakest position of full extension, and recruits all three heads.

The body has a number of protective neuromuscular reflexes to prevent injuries. It has been shown that pressure on the ulnar surface of the palm (little-finger side) causes an extensor or stabilization response in the triceps. This reflex allows greater contraction of the triceps. A technique called the triceps reflex extensor maneuver can be used in the bench press. The hands are positioned by internally rotating the arm five degrees when the person is under the bar, and the bar sits across the palm. This technique can also be used in the triceps push-down by internally rotating the hands on the bar and allowing the elbows to swing out. This powerlifter version of the push-down allows more contraction and strength development, especially of the long head.

Gorman states that the strength of the triceps, like that of the biceps, varies with the arm position relative to the shoulder. For example, if the arm is above the shoulder as in overhead triceps extension, triceps extension strength is 43 kilograms (95 pounds). If the arm is level with the shoulder as in horizontal machine triceps extension, triceps extension strength is 37 kilograms (82 pounds). If the arm is down to the side and pushing down, as in a dip, triceps extension strength is 51 kilograms (112 pounds). Triceps extension strength is greater with the arm below the shoulder than above it. That is why the dip is one of the better triceps exercises if the shoulders are healthy enough to do them.

Forearm Muscles

The forearm contains many muscles, but the three main ones are the brachioradialis, the extensor carpi radialis, and the flexor carpi radialis.

The brachioradialis arises from the upper two-thirds of the lateral supracondylar ridge of the humerus and inserts into the lateral styloid process of the radius. Its main function is flexing the elbow when the hand is in a neutral position (as in a thumb-up arm curl). It shows little activity in slow, easy flexion and is more active in rapid flexion and extension.

The extensor carpi radialis arises from the distal third of the lateral supracondylar ridge of the humerus and inserts into the second metacarpal on the back of the hand. Its main function is extension and abduction of the wrist, and it also aids in flexion of the forearm.

The flexor carpi radialis arises from the flexor tendon of the medial epicondyle of the humerus and inserts into the base of the second and third metacarpals of the hand. Its main function is flexion and abduction of the wrist, and it aids in pronation of the forearm.

Indications of Weakness

The forearm may become weak in a number of ways. One is through repetitive muscle trauma that causes the muscles to become shortened with adhesions. This is commonly known as tennis elbow, which causes pain on the outer (lateral) side of the elbow joint. Pain on the inner (medial) side of the elbow joint indicates that the forearm flexor muscles are also shortened with adhesions. If the proximal radioulnar (elbow) joint has restrictions, the forearm may also become weak and hard to pronate and supinate when lifting weight.

Optimal Training Principles

To train the brachioradialis, which is one of the larger muscles in the forearm, one of the best exercises is a reverse-grip E-Z bar curl. A pronated or semipronated (E-Z curl bar) grip puts the biceps at a mechanical disadvantage and increases the load on the brachioradialis and brachialis. The hammer curl is also an excellent exercise to train the brachioradialis and brachialis since the arm is in a semipronated position and there is less stress on the wrist than in reverse curls.

Dumbbell wrist extensions off a bench or the knee are an excellent way to develop strong wrist extensor muscles. A straight barbell can put excessive stress on the wrist joint potentially causing an injury. The dumbbell allows ulnar or radial deviation during wrist extension, thus working different wrist extensor muscles.

Wrist flexor muscles can be trained with barbell or dumbbell wrist curls, which use no pronation and place no stress on the wrist. To use heavier weight to load the muscles, use a barbell. To work various wrist flexor muscles, deviate the wrist radially or ulnarly on wrist flexion. To increase the stress on the flexor muscles at the top of the curl, change the angle: Instead of holding the forearms parallel to the floor, rest the arms at a 45-degree angle on top of the legs in a semistanding position, or use a preacher curl bench to change the end contraction position.

Upper-Back Muscles

The upper back is composed of: the trapezius (upper, middle, and lower), rhomboid, and latissimus dorsi. The upper trapezius muscle arises from the occiput, ligamentum nuchae, and the spinous process of the seventh cervical vertebra and inserts into the acromion process and the lateral third of the clavicle. Its main action is to elevate the shoulder and laterally flex the head and neck; it also assists in cervical extension.

The middle trapezius arises from the spinous processes of the sixth cervical to the third thoracic vertebrae and inserts into the acromion process and the spine of the scapula. The lower trapezius muscle arises from the spinous processes of the third to the twelfth thoracic vertebrae and inserts into medial aspect of the spine of the scapula. The function of middle and lower trapezius muscle is to assist in flexion and abduction of the humerus by rotating the glenoid cavity and to assist in maintaining a normal kyphotic posture in the upper thoracic spine.

The rhomboid muscle arises from the spinous processes of the seventh cervical to the fifth thoracic vertebrae and inserts into the medial border of the spine of the scapula. Its main action is to elevate and retract the scapula toward the spine and give stability to the scapula and shoulder. It also prevents winging of the scapula when the arm is lifting a weight.

The latissimus dorsi muscle arises from the thoracolumbar fascia, crest of the ilium, lower six thoracic vertebrae, and the last four ribs and inserts into the intertubercular groove of the humerus. Its main action is to depress the shoulder and extend the humerus, and it also adducts and assists in internal rotation of the humerus. Bilateral contraction of the latissimus dorsi assists in extension of the thoracic spine.

Indications of Weakness

Weakness in the upper trapezius muscle causes dropping of the shoulder on the affected side. If the muscles on both sides are weak, the head is anterior to the thoracic cage. Weakness of the middle trapezius muscle gives a round-shoulder appearance and causes forward protraction of the scapula. The thoracic spine may also have an increased kyphotic curve. Weakness of the latissimus dorsi allows the shoulder to elevate and move anteriorly in a standing posture. It may also cause difficulty in depressing the shoulder when the arm is overhead and pulling down.

Optimal Training Principles

The two main ways to train the upper back are to pull weights, cables, or body weight down from overhead (as in lat pulldowns or chin-ups) or to pull in toward the body from the front (as in rowing). There are many exercises that work different sections of the upper back.

To develop the upper trapezius, the best exercise is the dumbbell shrug. To do this exercise properly, the person must make sure that the dumbbells stay beside the body and do not drift forward causing torsion and shear on the acromioclavicular and sternoclavicular joints. The head should stay up at all times, and the person must resist the urge to put the chin down to get extra stretch because the risk of cervical disk injury increases when the cervical spine is flexed. The dumbbells should be raised as high as possible and then lowered. Rolling the shoulders has minimal effect on the trapezius.

To exercise the middle trapezius, the bent-over dumbbell laterals with the elbows in line with the shoulders will stress the posterior deltoid and middle trapezius.

To exercise the lower trapezius, the best exercise is the Superman exercise on the Swiss ball. The person should lie face down with the Swiss ball at the level of chest and abdomen and use just one arm at a time. The person starts with either the left arm at the 11:00 position or the right arm at the 1:00 position with the thumb up. The person lifts the arm until the trapezius is maximally contracted and then lowers the arm. The lower trapezius muscle is usually the weakest muscle in the upper back, and this abnormal muscle mechanics can cause upper-back pain and shoulder instability.

To exercise the rhomboid muscle maximally, the one-arm seated cable row exercise can be modified. Keeping the elbow at the same height as the shoulder, the person brings the elbow back until the hand is in line with the shoulder and then brings the arm and shoulder back as a unit to retract the scapula maximally. This increases the contraction of the rhomboid, a muscle that is usually not exercised much by people who sit in front of a keyboard with the shoulders forward. This excellent exercise helps increase the strength of the rhomboid and reduces pain between the shoulder blades when working at a computer.

The lat pulldown is an excellent all-around exercise for the latissimus dorsi. It has a few different versions, but the most effective is pulling the bar down to the top of the chest in the front. Another version is pulling the bar down behind the head to the base of the neck, which increases stress on the shoulder capsule and does not allow enough arm extension for maximal latissimus dorsi contraction. A useful technique when starting the exercise with full arm extension, is to allow the bar to rise until the shoulders also rise, then pull the shoulders down first without bending the arms, and finally bend the arms to pull the bar down to the chest. This allows increased range of motion and tension on the latissimus dorsi for increased strength and development.

The chin-up (palms facing toward the body) and pull-up (palms facing away) are excellent upper-back exercises. They work differently from the lat pull-down because they involve pulling the body up to the bar rather than pulling the bar down to the body. From a developmental and neurological standpoint, this is a more functional exercise that we use in everyday life. The style of chin-up dictates which muscles it focuses on. A narrow to medium grip while pulling the body up until the bar hits the chest stresses the upper latissimus dorsi and biceps. Using a V-bar with hands facing each other stresses the rhomboids and lower latissimus dorsi more. To stress the latissimus dorsi even more, on the descent the person can slowly lower him- or herself at about half the normal speed until halfway down and then push the elbows forward and externally rotate the arms while lowering to the bottom position. This external rotation of the humerus stresses the lower latissimus dorsi muscle to develop a longer, fuller back width.

Two versions of seated rowing stress different parts of the upper back. A palms-up or palms-inward grip with the arms close to the body tends to stress the latissimus dorsi and rhomboids due to the amount of arm extension that can be achieved as the bar is pulled in toward the abdomen. An overhand grip with the elbows kept at shoulder height works the posterior deltoid, mid-trapezius, and rhomboid more as the bar is pulled in toward the chest.

To work the rhomboid more effectively, an alternative way to do the one-arm dumbbell row is to position the upper arm at 90 degrees to the body, instead of close to the body, with the palm facing backward while pulling up. Pulling the arm up all the way and then retracting the whole arm and shoulder maximally contracts the rhomboid muscle.

Lower-Back and Hip Muscles

The lower back and hips have many muscles, but the main ones involved in lifting are the lumbar erector spinae, psoas, quadratus lumborum, gluteus maximus, gluteus medius, and tensor fasciae latae.

The lumbar erector spinae arises from the iliac crest and thoracolumbar fascia and inserts into the lower thoracic ribs and the transverse and spinous processes of the lumbar vertebrae. Contraction of the lumbar erector spinae extends the trunk, and contraction on one side only assists in lateral lumbar flexion. EMG studies show no activity of the erector spinae in full lumbar flexion; it is relaxed when the lumbar spine flexes.

The psoas arises from the vertebral bodies and disks of the twelfth thoracic to the fifth lumbar vertebrae and inserts into the lesser trochanter of the femur. The psoas flexes the femur on the pelvis and also flexes the trunk on the pelvis.

The quadratus lumborum arises from the posterior iliac crest and inserts into the transverse processes of the first to fourth lumbar vertebrae and into twelfth rib. The quadratus lumborum lifts the legs if the upper body is held down in one position on its side. It also laterally bends the lumbar spine and lifts the upper body if the pelvis is held down in one position on its side. The quadratus lumborum helps support the pelvis and the lumbar spine.

The gluteus maximus arises from the posterior ilium, iliac crest, sacrum, and sacrotuberous ligament and inserts into the gluteal tuberosity of the femur and iliotibial band of the tensor fasciae latae. The gluteus maximus extends and laterally rotates the thigh, aids in abduction of the thigh, and maximally contracts during walking with long strides.

The gluteus medius arises from the ilium and anterior iliac crest and inserts into the greater tuberosity of the femur. The gluteus medius is the primary abductor of the femur and assists in medial rotation of the thigh.

The tensor fasciae latae arises from the anterior iliac crest and iliac spine and inserts into the lateral patellar retinaculum and lateral tibia. The tensor fasciae latae assists in thigh flexion, abduction, and medial rotation.

Indications of Weakness

Weakness of the lumbar erector spinae decreases lumbar extension strength and causes instability of the lumbar vertebrae. Chronic contraction of the muscle can also cause spinal curvature of the lumbar spine, potentially creating pain in the facet joints.

Weak hamstrings can increase hypertonicity in the lumbar erector spinae because the ilia are allowed to rotate anteriorly, increasing lumbar lordosis and jamming the lumbar facet joints.

If the psoas on one side is weak, walking stride is shortened on the weak side. If the psoas on both sides are weak, the lumbar spine is destabilized, and there may be pain in the region of the inguinal ligament.

If the quadratus lumborum is weak, lumbar flexion can cause muscle spasms. Over time, shortening of the quadratus lumborum creates a jamming of the facet joints, called imbrication, and causes pain during lumbar extension or exercises with axial load such as the squat or dead lift.

Weakness of the gluteus maximus makes it difficult to rise out of a chair; the hands are needed to push off the armrests. It may also cause lateral knee instability when the knee is loaded during squats or dead lifts. If the gluteus maximus is shortened and hypertonic, there may be increased lumbar lordosis with potential scoliosis on the affected side.

If the gluteus medius muscle is weak, a standing posture exam reveals that the ilium is higher on the side of weakness. Leg abduction strength is also decreased and there is pain in the area of the gluteus medius when squatting.

Tensor fasciae latae weakness causes pain in the hip and lateral knee area and decreases lateral knee support while flexing the knee, as in squatting or running. This combination of dysfunctions is called iliotibial band syndrome or snapping hip syndrome.

Optimal Training Principles

The main exercise for the lower back and hips is the dead lift. This movement is used everyday for picking objects up off the floor. The dead lift is one of the best ways to learn how to lift. The erector spinae is one of the main muscles responsible for lumbar extension in the dead lift, but to get a weight off the floor, knowing how and when to use the feet and legs is also necessary. When starting the lift, the person should sit back on the heels and visualize driving them through the floor. This technique makes the person start with the legs and also prevents the person's weight from shifting from the heels onto the balls of the feet and big toe. If the person allows the weight to shift onto the balls of the feet and big toe, the feet may pronate excessively, causing the interphalangeal joints and muscles of the feet to stretch. This in turn causes abnormal proprioception of the foot, which may inhibit the hip and back extensor muscles. Janda, a neurologist, did some research on volunteers where he increased the arch in the foot by putting an arch in the shoe and he also put a small ball on the bottom of the shoe to make it unstable to exercise the foot and ankle for increased proprioception. After two weeks of the volunteers walking around with this shoe, he measured a 200 percent increase in the speed of contraction of the gluteus maximus and medius because of the increased proprioception from the foot. Proper footwear with good arches helps the person functionally and neurologically in their lifts.

The person should start the dead lift with the bar as close to the body as possible. This decreases the length of the lever to make the biomechanics more favorable. Allowing the bar to swing out away from the legs dramatically increases the strength needed to lift the weight.

When performing the basic extension exercise, the person should be sure to extend the lumbar erector spinae during the ascent phase and to curl the upper body and spine to increase lumbar flexion when returning the start position. This flexion and extension of the lumbar spine increases the magnitude of erector spinae contractions.

The reverse hyper machine exercise popularized by powerlifter and coach Louie Simmons is excellent for increasing the strength of the lower back and hips. The reverse hyper involves raising the legs with weight to horizontal while the torso is supported by a bench. It works the gluteus maximus, hamstrings, and lumbar erector spinae without putting any axial load on the spine. The start position of the reverse hyper simulates the beginning of a dead lift, where the back is lengthened; raising the legs by increased contraction of the gluteus maximus simulates the lockout position of the dead lift.

Quadriceps Femoris Muscles

The quadriceps femoris muscle group is made of up four muscles: the rectus femoris, vastus lateralis, vastus intermedius, and vastus medialis.

The rectus femoris arises from the anteroinferior iliac spine and the brim of the acetabulum and inserts into the superior surface of the patella along with the fibers of the vastus muscles; the inferior patellar ligament then inserts into the tibial tubercle. The rectus femoris crosses two joints, the hip and the knee, so it has varied functions. The rectus femoris extends the lower leg and assists in flexing the thigh on the pelvis; when the thigh is fixed, it helps flex the trunk on the thigh. The rectus femoris provides only one-fifth of the total force of the quadriceps and cannot fully extend the knee by itself. The vastus muscles, especially the medialis, synergistically assist in full knee extension.

The vastus lateralis arises from the greater trochanter, gluteal tuberosity, and lateral aspect of the upper three-fourths of the femur and inserts into the superior surface of the patella along with the fibers of the other vastus muscles; the inferior patellar ligament then inserts into the tibial tubercle. The vastus lateralis is the largest quadriceps muscle and crosses only one joint. It extends the lower leg and helps stabilize the knee joint, along with the medialis.

The vastus intermedius arises from the anterior and lateral two-thirds of the upper femur and inserts into the superior surface of the patella along with the fibers of the other vastus muscles; the inferior patellar ligament then inserts into the tibial tubercle. The vastus intermedius crosses one joint and extends the lower leg.

The vastus medialis arises from the posteromedial femur and the tendons of the adductor longus and magnus and inserts into the superior surface of the patella along with the fibers of the other vastus muscles; the inferior patellar ligament then inserts into the tibial tubercle. The lowest fibers, the vastus medialis oblique (VMO), are almost horizontal and contract maximally during the final stage of knee extension to retain the patella in the patellar groove of the femur.

Indications of Weakness

General weakness of the rectus femoris on one side may result in posterior rotation of the ilium. When the clinician or trainer assesses hip levels by putting his or her hands on the top of the standing athlete's ilium, the pelvis appears relatively low on the side of weakness. Weakness of the vastus lateralis or medialis muscle manifests as an abnormal position or motion of the patella with chronic instability of the knee. There can be pain under the patella if the quadriceps are shortened and too tight, thus compressing the patella abnormally into the patellar groove.

Optimal Training Principles

Compound movements for training the quadriceps, such as the squat and leg press, should be used first to enhance the normal movement patterns of the body before performing isolated single-joint exercises, such as leg extensions.

Deep barbell squats in which the thighs are below parallel to the ground, strengthen the vastus medialis oblique (VMO), which is responsible for full knee extension and stability. Deep squats activate the VMO more than regular squats or leg extension and help stabilize the knee.

Rotating the lower leg internally (pointing the toes in) on a leg extension machine increases the stress on the vastus lateralis. Externally rotating the lower leg (pointing the toes out) focuses on the vastus medialis. To stress the rectus femoris, extend the upper body on the leg extension machine to posteriorly tilt the pelvis and thus stretch the rectus femoris more.

If the anterior cruciate ligament (ACL) has been injured and surgically repaired, the person should refrain from performing any leg extension. Leg extensions contract the quadriceps and pull the tibia anteriorly, which puts undue stress on the ACL ligament and might injure it again. Instead, the person can perform the squat or leg press; the axial load of these exercises causes a co-contraction of the quadriceps and hamstrings and thus decreases anterior tension on the tibia and allows the ACL to heal properly.

Two variations of the squat focus on different parts of the legs. A closer stance with increased knee flexion, often referred to as the bodybuilding squat, offers more quadriceps development. The person starts the exercise by first pushing the knees forward, moving into a deep squatting position, and then coming back up. This puts maximum stress on the quadriceps. To increase strength, the person takes a wider than shoulder-width stance with the feet turned out 10 degrees and starts the descent while shifting the weight onto the heels, pushing back the hips, and keeping the arch in the back. The person should keep the knees over the ankles, descend until the thighs are below parallel with the ground, and then drive the hips forward during the ascent. This variation, often referred to as the powerlifting squat, builds explosive strength in the hip and gluteal region with some stress on the quadriceps.

Hamstring Muscles

The hamstring muscle group is made of up three separate muscles: the biceps femoris, the semimembranosus, and the semitendinosus.

The biceps femoris, known as the lateral hamstring, has a long head and a short head. The long head arises from the ischial tuberosity and sacrotuberous ligament and inserts into the lateral side of the fibula and tibia. The long head crosses both the hip joint and knee joint. When contracted, it extends the thigh and flexes the knee. The short head arises from the lateral side of the femur and inserts into the lateral side of the fibula and tibia. This means that the short head crosses only the knee joint and is involved only in flexing the knee. Both heads laterally rotate the foot outward when the knee is semiflexed.

The semimembranosus and semitendinosus muscles are known as the medial hamstrings. They both arise from the ischial tuberosity, cross the hip and the knee joints, and insert into the medial tibia. They are both involved in extending the thigh, flexing the knee, and medially rotating the foot inward.

Indications of Weakness

General weakness of the hamstrings on one side may result in an anterior rotation of the innominate bone. When the clinician or trainer assesses hip levels by putting his or her hands on the top of the standing person's ilium, the pelvis appears relatively high on the side of weakness. Weakness of the medial hamstrings can result in the development of genu varum (bowleg) due to lateral rotation of the thigh and tibia. Weakness of the lateral hamstrings can result in genu valgum (knock-knee) due to medial rotation of the thigh and tibia. Hamstring curls with the feet turned in or out may help remedy these dysfunctions.

Optimal Training Principles

The hamstrings have two major functions, knee flexion and thigh extension, so it is important to train both movements by using different types of exercise. Seated, prone, and standing leg curl machines strengthen knee flexion by working both heads of the biceps femoris along with the semitendinosus and semimembranosus muscles. Exercises such as Romanian dead lifts, good mornings, back extensions, and reverse hyperextensions strengthen hip extension and work the long head of the biceps along with the semitendinosus and semimembranosus muscles.

The person can rotate the feet outward to focus more stress on the lateral hamstrings and rotate the feet inward to increase the stress on the medial hamstrings. Keeping the feet pointing straight forward stresses both heads equally. Plantar-flexing the feet (pointing the toes) increases the stress on the hamstrings and decreases the synergistic involvement of the gastrocnemius as a knee flexor.

Hamstrings are predominantly fast-twitch muscles and respond well to fewer (less than 10) repetitions and more weight for strength and muscular development.

Calf Muscles

The calf muscle group is made up of two separate muscles: the gastrocnemius and soleus. The gastrocnemius, or calf muscle, arises from the medial and lateral condyles of the femur and inserts into the achilles tendon, which attaches to the calcaneus. Its main action is plantar flexion of the foot, and it assists in flexion of the knee. The gastrocnemius is the third most powerful muscle in the body after the gluteus maximus and quadriceps femoris. When the knee is fully extended, the gastrocnemius is passively stretched and works at its best advantage. When the knee is flexed, gastrocnemius tension decreases, and the muscle loses its strength efficiency.

The soleus muscle arises from the head of the fibula and the posterior surface of the tibia and joins with the fibers of the gastrocnemius to insert into the achilles tendon where it attaches to the calcaneus. Its main action is plantar flexion of the foot. EMG of the soleus shows continuous activity in all positions of the knee during running, climbing, and jumping, but its power is inadequate compared with the gastrocnemius.

Indications of Weakness

When the calf is weakened, a person stands with an anterior lean since the calf does not have enough strength to keep the body upright. The inability to rise on the toes is commonly seen after surgery for a ruptured achilles tendon.

Optimal Training Principles

A standing calf raise with the knee fully extended on the ascent and descent exercises the gastrocnemius maximally. This ensures that the gastrocnemius is under full tension for maximum strength. To exercise the soleus maximally, the knee has to be bent at least 90 degrees to take the tension out of the gastrocnemius.

Rising up on the big toe during the ascent in the standing calf raise exercises the calf more effectively and efficiently. This activates the flexor hallucis longus and brevis, which flexes the big toe and assist in plantar flexion also.

A discovery by bodybuilder Larry Scott explains why the donkey calf raise is such a great calf exercise: the hamstrings circle around the outside and under the heads of the gastrocnemius before its attachment to the lower leg. That is why bending over at the waist increases the tension on the hamstrings and makes the calves tighter. The more tension on the gastrocnemius, the stronger it becomes. This is why the donkey calf raise is so effective.

Changing the foot position exercises various muscles of the calf. Turning the toes inward forces some inversion and stresses the tibialis posterior, which is on the inside of the calf. Pointing the toes outward forces some eversion and exercises the peroneal muscle group on the outside of the calf. Although it is commonly said that turning the feet in or out develops the medial or lateral gastrocnemius, it is actually the tibialis posterior and peroneal muscles that are stressed more.

Abdominal Muscles

The abdominal muscle group is composed of three muscles: the rectus abdominis, the abdominal oblique, and the transversus abdominis.

The rectus abdominis arises from the symphysis pubis and crest of the pubis and inserts into the costal cartilage of the fifth, sixth, and seventh ribs and into the lateral aspects of the xiphoid process. The rectus abdominis flexes the spine on the pelvis, supports the abdominal viscera, and aids in anterior support for the pelvis.

The abdominal oblique arises from the ninth to twelfth ribs and inserts into the lateral surface of the iliac crest. The abdominal oblique rotates and laterally flexes the spine on the pelvis and also supports the abdominal viscera.

The transversus abdominis arises from the inguinal ligament, the iliac crest, the lumbothoracic fascia, and the lower six ribs, and then the fibers run horizontally to attach into the linea alba. The transversus abdominis supports the abdominal viscera and aids in rotational support of the pelvis.

Indications of Weakness

Anterior abdominal weakness causes chronic instability of the pelvis due to abnormal pelvic rotation and movement. Weakness of the abdominal muscles can be identified by potting of the upper or lower abdominal wall.

Shortening of the rectus abdominis can increase thoracic kyphosis and cause the head to be carried anteriorly. This in turn can decrease cervical and thoracic rotation and cause pain and discomfort in the region of the cervical and thoracic spine.

If the transversus abdominis is weak, the abdomen relaxes at 70 degrees of lumbar flexion. This decreases the tension on the thoracolumbar fascia and the stability of the lumbar and pelvic region.

Optimal Training Principles

The abdominals are optimally trained in different movement patterns that increase stability, strength, and muscular development. To strengthen and work the rectus abdominis, the person needs to flex or curl the spine while lying on the floor until the abdominals are maximally contracted, an exercise known as the abdominal crunch. Taking and holding a deep breath during the set triggers a little-known reflex that neurologically inhibits the rectus abdominis and abdominal oblique muscles. Crunches should therefore be performed during expiration. Conventional sit-ups with the feet anchored down simulate the gait pattern at heel contact. This technique of foot fixation increases the activity in the tibialis anterior, quadriceps, and iliopsoas in a pattern called flexor synergy. This pattern can increase hyperextension of the lumbar spine with a possible increase in risk of injury. Keep the feet unanchored, and allow the abdominals to do the work.

Summary

To exercise muscles for strength and development, both great technique and an awareness of how the exercise affects the muscles in the body are important. Many exercise techniques are good, but the small changes explained in this chapter make them optimal. The next chapter examines the risks and benefits associated with specific variations in exercise techniques.

4

Analyzing the Risk–Benefit Ratio of Weight-Training Exercises

Along with a good understanding of muscle biomechanics, knowing how muscles function in weight-training exercises is also important. This knowledge enables the selection of the optimal technique while decreasing the risk of injury.

Starting a weight-training program is similar to undertaking other types of physical fitness activities. All fitness activities carry a risk. The risk depends on the activity, the equipment, the environment, the athlete's level of expertise, focus, conditioning, level of fatigue, the state of the athlete's tissues, previous injuries, and biomechanical factors. A coding system should be created to indicate the level of difficulty relative to the person's experience and needs to avoid injuries.

Certain sports, such as downhill skiing, surfing, and boating, have an established system of coding the level of difficulty to allow people to decide the activity risk based on their self-assessed experience level. For example, in downhill skiing, ski trails or runs are marked with colors and shapes as follows: green circles indicate the easiest beginner trails that present a low difficulty level and risk of injury, blue squares mark intermediate trails with a medium difficulty level and risk of injury, and black-diamond runs are for advanced and expert skiers and present a high difficulty level and risk of injury.

Each level also offers a certain level of enjoyment, personal satisfaction, and accomplishment, known as the benefit of skiing. Black-diamond trails have the highest potential benefit, blue-square trails have a medium potential benefit, and green-circle trails have low potential benefit for the skier to aspire to. A beginner skier belongs on the green runs. If he or she takes a black-diamond run, the risk of being injured is high. But an advanced skier can go down the same black-diamond run with minimal risk of injury because of his or her higher skill level and get the benefit of a sense of adventure and fun. The advanced skier may find a low-risk green run too easy and thus derive less benefit of excitement from it.

Risk–Benefit Coding System

A coding system for weight training allows the weightlifter to determine whether a certain volume, intensity, and technique will be of benefit and at what risk. Certain techniques offer a large benefit but also carry a large risk, but if the person's expertise is high enough, the trade-off may be worthwhile and can be done safely similar to the skiing example. **It is important to remember that high risk does not automatically mean that the person will be injured.** It means that the potential for injury may be higher due to specific techniques or training intensities needed for increased strength or development. A conditioned and experienced person with great technique and a properly functioning musculoskeletal system will lower this risk of injury. High-intensity training and volume always carry more risk than low intensity training and volume. The benefits gained from low-intensity training and volume is less for the experienced weight trainer.

The following coding system was developed to help individuals make decisions about the appropriate volume, intensity, and technique for weight-training programs.

1. Low Risk, Low Benefit

This is a great level for a beginner but not for an advanced lifter, unless he or she is going through an active-rest phase of recovery.

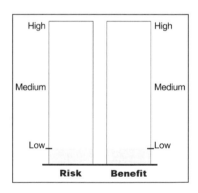

2. Medium Risk, Low Benefit

This level usually denotes a poor training technique or inappropriate training intensity with minimal benefit. It may not cause injury, but the benefits are minimal.

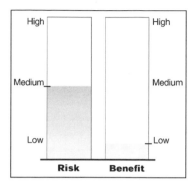

3. High Risk, Low Benefit

This level usually denotes a very poor training technique or inappropriate training intensity with minimal benefit. The potential of risk outweighs the benefit.

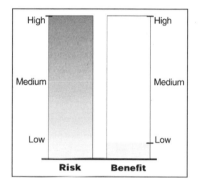

4. Low Risk, Medium Benefit

This is a great level for a beginner and possibly for an advanced lifter who is in an active-conditioning phase of training. This usually denotes good training technique with minimal potential risk.

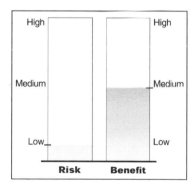

5. Low Risk, High Benefit

This is the best level to train at. It is great training technique and provides the highest benefits with minimal risk.

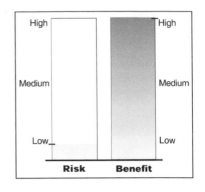

6. Medium Risk, Medium Benefit

This level usually denotes an increased training intensity and volume or using a more advanced technique which increases the benefits, but may also increase the risk of injury dependent on the experience and conditioning of the person. Proper monitoring of the body and recovery at this level is important to minimize risk.

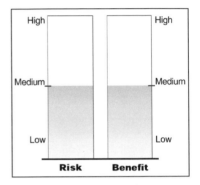

7. High Risk, Medium Benefit

This level usually denotes a poor training technique or inappropriate training intensity. The potential risk is high with only moderate benefit. Proper monitoring of the body and recovery at this level is important to minimize risk.

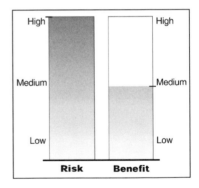

8. Medium Risk, High Benefit

This level usually denotes an increased train-ing intensity and volume or using a more advanced technique at an appropriate experience level for maximum benefit with moderate risk. Proper monitoring of the body and recovery at this level is important to minimize risk.

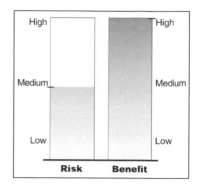

9. High Risk, High Benefit

This level usually denotes an increased training intensity and volume or using a more advanced technique at an advanced experience level with near maximum effort. This level is usually seen at the end stage of training for competition and also competi-tion lifting. Proper monitoring of the body and recovery at this level is very important to minimize risk.

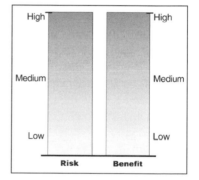

Variables That Affect the Risk–Benefit Ratio

Many variables that determine the risk benefit ratio of a weight-training program have to be considered. In general, the older the person, the higher the risk and the lower the benefit in strength and development due to decreased hormone levels and recuperation capabilities. Taller people with longer limbs and torsos have potentially higher risks due to poorer mechanical leverage which can increase the stress on the body. Movements further away from the body also can increase the stress on the joints and muscles.

Performing a Risk–Benefit Analysis

■ **Step 1—Determine the person's experience:** beginner (0–3 months of train-ing), intermediate (3–12 months), or advanced (over 12 months).

Less-experienced people should use low volume, intensity, and weight to allow body tissues such as ligaments and tendons to adapt to the stress of training. Experience also determines the speed of the exercise performed. The more experienced the person, the more explosive the lifting can be. Experience level also determines the volume of exercise for each body part and the amount of weight used.

■ **Step 2—Determine the desired outcome.**

Does the person want to increase muscle size or strength? Different types of training create different effects; choose the appropriate training load, volume, and exercise for the desired effect. Choose the most appropriate exercise techniques discussed at the end of this chapter for either muscle hypertrophy or strength. Choose the exercise technique with the highest amount of benefit and the least amount of risk that will give you your desired outcome. The heavier the weight lifted, the less the volume should be done to permit recovery from the training session.

■ **Step 3—Assess individual biomechanics.**

Is the person tall in height with long arms and legs or short in height with short arms and legs? Longer limbs make longer levers and may put more stress on the body. Exercises such as the dumbbell fly and lateral raise, in which the arms are outstretched away from the body, may put more stress on the joints due to the longer levers than the dumbbell bench press or dumbbell shoulder press.

If the person has a long torso and short legs, he or she may have difficulty remaining upright when squatting due to the long lever of the back. Such people can either wear lifting boots with a raised heel to lengthen the leg to or do front squats or leg presses to decrease the long lever effect.

Certain lifting techniques can also be modified to shift the stress to other muscle groups. For example, if the person has weak legs and strong hips in the squat and is interested in increasing his or her strength, the squat style can be changed to be less upright in the trunk with the lower leg remaining vertical throughout the lift. This will reduce the stress around the knee and leg muscles by increasing the horizontal distance from the low back with less knee flexion, which increases the stress on the hip joint and the gluteal and hamstring muscles.

To lift the maximum amount of weight in lifts such as the dead lift or power clean, make sure that the bar stays within a few inches of the body at all times. This decreases the leverage stress on the lower back. For example, if a 20-kilogram (44-pound) weight is eight inches from the body, the resultant force on the lumbar spine is 120 kilograms (265 pounds). If the same weight is 12 inches from the body, the resultant force increases to 160 kilograms (353 pounds), an increase in the resultant force on the lumbar spine of 40 kilograms (88 pounds) for a four-inch difference in distance. Keep the weight close to the body at all times to decrease the stress on the lower back to minimize injury.

■ **Step 4—Assess the body's structural alignment.**

Any structural aberrations such as scoliosis or a structurally short leg can change body alignment when lifting. With a large deviation of the spine such as scoliosis, a heavy axial load as in the squat can unduly stress the spine and the specific joints at the regions of maximum curvature in the inexperienced trainer, potentially causing the torso to twist on the ascent. A solution is to do leg presses or machine squats instead, which diminish torquing and twisting until the body is strong enough to do freehand squats. For a person with a structurally short leg, a lift in the shoe can lengthen the leg to match the other, or the person can use open-chain exercises such as the leg extension or leg curl rather than closed-chain exercises such as the squat or leg press.

Risk-Benefit Ratio of Volume and Intensity

Reviewing general principles of how volume and intensity affect the beginning, intermediate, and advanced weight trainer gives a guideline for program design.

Beginner Training Level

At the beginner level of training (0–3 months), it is best to use more repetitions, fewer sets, and lower weights. The first few months of training conditions the body for stress during training. If stress is increased too fast during this first stage, injuries such as strains, sprains, and myofasciitis may occur needlessly. It is better to go more slowly at the beginning of the training program to develop proper neural programming of exercise technique for maximum strength and development.

Volume and intensity for the beginner should be low enough to allow proper recuperation but still enough stimulus for increasing strength and growth. For low risk and low benefit, do one to two sets per body part of 12 or more reps at 65 percent or less of the one-repetition maximum (1RM). This is a good starting level for the first few weeks for beginners to learn the exercise movements.

For low risk and medium benefit, perform three to four sets per body part of 12 or more reps at 65 percent or less of 1RM. The volume can increase from one to two sets, to three sets after the initial few weeks for greater stress on the muscles. Another choice for low risk and medium benefit is fewer sets, one to two per body part, of 6 to 12 reps at an increased intensity of 67 to 85 percent of 1RM. The intensity (weight) can be increased after the initial few weeks.

Five or more sets per body part of 12 or more reps at 65 percent or less of 1RM offer a medium risk with a medium benefit. Another combination for medium risk with medium benefit is increasing the volume and intensity to three to five sets per body part of 6 to 12 reps at 67 to 85 percent of 1RM. The increased volume and intensity can be implemented four to eight weeks after starting a program and requires monitoring of how well the person recovers to determine if it may be too much stress.

Training intensity of one to five reps at 85 to 100 percent 1RM offers a high risk and is inappropriate for a beginner whose muscles and ligaments are not conditioned to handle the heavy load.

Intermediate Training Level

The intermediate level, 3 to 12 months of training, is when a lot of strength and muscular development occurs if the program is good and the person stays injury-free. The number of sets and intensity can increase and the number of reps decrease to produce gains in strength and development.

At this level, one to two sets per body part of 12 or more reps at 65 percent or less of 1RM offers low risk with low benefit. One to two sets per body part of 6 to 12 reps at 67 to 85 percent of 1RM also offers low risk with low benefit. The volume and intensity may be too low for any progress in strength and development.

Three or more sets per body part of 12 or more reps at 65 percent or less of 1RM offer low risk with medium benefit. The increased volume increases stress on the muscles, which can be done after the initial few months of training. The amount by which volume can increase after the initial months depends on the person's recovery capacity and size of body part. The larger the body part, the greater the volume possible.

Three to four sets per body part of 6 to 12 reps at 67 to 85 percent of 1RM also offers low risk with medium benefit. The increased volume and intensity, which depend on the recovery capacity of the person and size of body part, stress the body enough for potential increases in strength and development.

A volume increase to five or more sets per body part of 6 to 12 reps at 67 to 85 percent of 1RM offers medium risk with high benefit. The increased volume and intensity, which depend on the recovery capacity of the person and size of body part, stress the body enough for potential increases in strength and development.

If the volume is reduced to one to two sets per body part of one to five reps and the intensity increased to 85 to 100 percent of 1RM, there is medium risk with medium benefit. The increased intensity with low volume mildly increases the injury risk but potentially increases strength more then the previous intensity level. Muscles and ligaments may not be conditioned enough to handle a heavy weight with high intensity and requires monitoring of how well the person recovers to determine if it may be too much stress.

Three to four sets per body part of one to five reps at 85 to 100 percent of 1RM offers medium risk with medium benefit. The increased volume moderately increases the injury risk while it potentially also increases strength. Muscles and ligaments may not be conditioned to handle the heavy load and requires monitoring of how well the person recovers to determine if it may be too much stress.

Five or more sets per body part of one to five reps at 85 to 100 percent of 1RM offer high risk with medium benefit. The increased volume severely increases the injury risk with potential increases of strength. Muscles and ligaments may not be conditioned to handle the heavy load and volume and requires monitoring of how well the person recovers to determine if it may be too much stress.

Advanced Training Level
The advanced training level, over 12 months, is when training can start to focus more intensely on strength or muscular development. At this level, periodization can be utilized to continually alter the amount of training stress up and down over a period of months allowing the body to recuperate and stay injury-free. The number of sets and repetitions can increase to produce gains of strength and development.

One to two sets per body part of 12 or more reps at 65 percent or less of 1RM and 6 to 12 reps at an increased intensity of 67 to 85 percent of 1RM offer low risk with low benefit. The volume and intensity are too low for increased strength and development in an advanced lifter. This is a good level for active rest for an advanced lifter who is recovering from a competition.

Three to four sets per body part of 12 or more reps at 65 percent or less of 1RM offer low risk with medium benefit. The volume and intensity level may be too low for increased strength and development for the advanced lifter. Sets of 15 to 30 reps may make for a good muscular endurance session.

Five or more sets per body part of 12 or more reps at 65 percent or less of 1RM offer low risk with high benefit. The increased volume and low intensity are good for endurance training. The gains depends on the person's recovery capacity, the size of the body part, and training effect wanted.

Three to four sets per body part of 6 to 12 reps at 67 to 85 percent of 1RM offer low risk with medium benefit. The volume and intensity offer a good balance between muscle hypertrophy and strength.

Five or more sets per body part of 6 to 12 reps at 67 to 85 percent of 1RM offer medium risk with high benefit. The volume and intensity offer a good balance between muscle hypertrophy and strength training.

A decreased volume of one to two sets per body part of one to five reps at an increased intensity of 85 to 100 percent of 1RM offers medium risk with medium benefit. The increased intensity mildly increases the injury risk but may increase strength and muscular hypertrophy more.

Increasing the volume to three to four sets per body part of one to five reps at 85 to 100 percent of 1RM offers medium risk with high benefit. The high intensity with increased volume mildly increases the injury risk but also makes possible larger increases in strength and some muscle hypertrophy. Muscles and ligaments may not be able to handle the heavy load with increased volume; the body's ability to handle this load and volume depends on training and genetics.

Increasing the volume to five or more sets per body part of one to five reps at 85 to 100 percent of 1RM offers high risk with high benefit. The high intensity with increased volume severely increases the injury risk, but also large gains in strength may be developed if the person can recover from the training sessions.

Risk–Benefit Ratio of Weight-Training Exercise Parameters

Certain weight-training exercise parameters carry more risk than others. General parameters of weight training include speed, control, stability, tightness, head position, and breathing. Any modification of these parameters changes the risk–benefit ratio. Always choose the parameter with the highest benefit and the least risk, except for experienced lifters trying to get a specific result.

■ A controlled movement pattern at slow to medium speed offers low risk with medium benefit; this is a good way for beginners to perfect their exercise technique.

■ A controlled movement pattern at medium to fast speed offers low risk with medium benefit. Explosive but controlled speed increases strength. These combinations can be used by either intermediate or advanced trainers.

■ An uncontrolled movement pattern at fast speed carries a high risk with low benefits. The lack of control with excessive speed can injure tissues by overloading them.

- A stable and tight position during exercise offers low risk with medium benefit. This is a good way for beginners to perfect their exercise technique.

- An unstable or loose position during exercise carries medium risk with medium benefit. Unstable surfaces such as wobble boards or stability balls with light weights can increase proprioception for better neurological control. Lack of tightness with heavy weights may cause improper technique and increase risk of injury.

- An exercise position that is both unstable and loose offers a high risk with no benefit. Lack of stability and tightness with heavy weights may cause improper technique and increase risk of injury.

- Keeping the head straight when lifting offers low risk with low benefit. This is the proper position for the head and results in normal stress on the cervical muscles and vertebral disks.

- Flexing the neck forward carries medium risk with low benefit. Neck flexion increases the stress on the cervical muscles, ligaments, and disks.

- Flexing the neck forward and holding the breath while lifting carries a high risk with low benefit. Neck flexion along with increasing interthoracic pressure may cause cervical disk herniation.

- Inhaling during the exertion portion of a repetition offers low risk with low benefit. This decreases the interthoracic pressure and thus stress on the disks, but it also decreases force production when lifting the weight.

- Exhaling during the exertion portion of the repetition offers medium risk with medium benefit. It increases interthoracic pressure, which increases risk to the vertebral disks, but it is also increases force production so that more weight can be lifted.

- Holding the breath during a set carries high risk with medium benefit. It severely increases interthoracic pressure, which increases risk to the vertebral disks, and also increases the possibility of passing out. The benefit is increased force production for lifting more weight, but only for a few reps.

Risk–Benefit Ratio of Specific Weight-Training Exercise Techniques

Each weight-training exercise can be performed in various ways. Some techniques are beneficial for the development of strength, while other techniques are more suited for muscular hypertrophy. The benefit and inherent risk of each exercise modification such as grip width, foot position, arm position, range of motion, head position, and trunk motion will alter dependent on the person's experience, body type, and outcomes desired. The exercise modifications should always be done to increase the stress on the muscles and not the joints, ligaments, or capsules. The following pages review variations in technique for each weight-training exercise to offer guidelines for the optimal implementation in an individual training program. Remember that high risk does not automatically mean that the person will be injured. It means that the potential for injury may be higher due to specific techniques needed for increased strength and development

Barbell bench press *Medium-width hand grip*

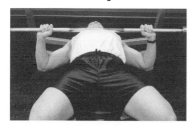 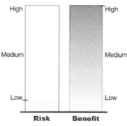

This technique keeps the forearm perpendicular to the floor at the bottom with minimal wrist stress.

Barbell bench press *Wide hand grip*

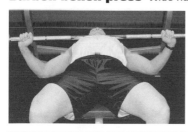 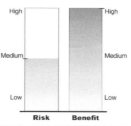

The wrist is under stress because of the angle of the forearm. The benefit is a shorter arm stroke for potentially lifting more weight.

Barbell bench press *Midchest contact point*

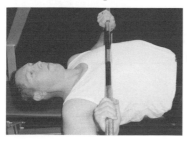 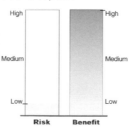

This is the most common and effective contact point of the bar on the chest.

Barbell bench press *High-chest contact point*

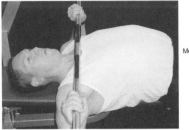

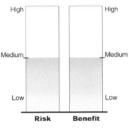

Risk | Benefit

The risk is increased stress on the shoulder capsule and A/C joint. The benefit is a small increase in stress on the upper pectoral muscle.

Barbell bench press *Upper arm at 45 degrees to body (at 4:00 and 8:00)*

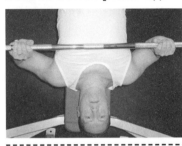

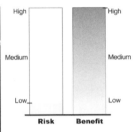

Risk | Benefit

The benefit is increased power with decreased stress on the shoulder joint and capsule. This is commonly called the powerlifting style.

Barbell bench press *Upper arm at 90 degrees to body (at 3:00 and 9:00)*

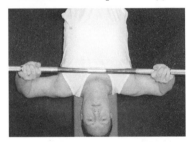

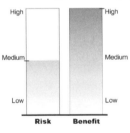

Risk | Benefit

The risk is increased stress on the shoulder capsule. The benefit is increased stress on the pectoral muscles. This is commonly called the bodybuilding style.

Barbell bench press *Raising hips off the bench during ascent*

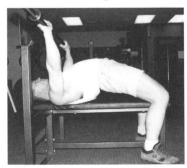

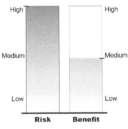

Risk | Benefit

The risk is increased stress on the low-back joints. The benefit is recovering from a technique flaw when the person allows the bar to bounce and go over the abdomen instead of the chest during ascent. The person tries to recover by changing the bar ascent angle by pushing up the hips to assist in pushing the bar back toward the chest.

Barbell bench press *Wrists hyperextended when pressing*

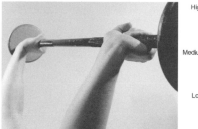

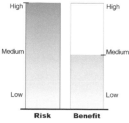

High
Medium
Low
Risk

High
Medium
Low
Benefit

The risk is increased stress on the wrist joint, which can potentially injure the metacarpal bones in the wrist. Wrist hyperextension risk is diminished with individuals who have small hands and large wrists, which reduces the leverage and stress on the joints.

Barbell bench press *Wrists straight when pressing*

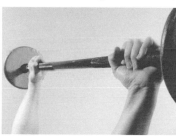

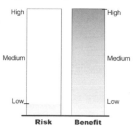

High
Medium
Low
Risk

High
Medium
Low
Benefit

The benefits are decreased stress on the wrist joint and more control on the bar as it is being pushed up.

Flat dumbbell fly *Elbows unlocked and upper arm parallel to the floor*

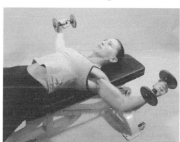

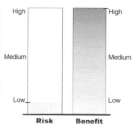

High
Medium
Low
Risk

High
Medium
Low
Benefit

The benefit is that the chest muscles are stressed adequately without overloading the shoulder joint and capsule.

Flat dumbbell fly *Elbows locked and upper arm parallel to the floor*

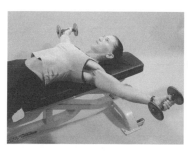

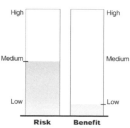

High
Medium
Low
Risk

High
Medium
Low
Benefit

The risk is increased stress on the shoulder joint and capsule and elbow joint. There is minimal benefit.

Flat dumbbell fly *Elbows unlocked and upper arm excessively below parallel to the floor*

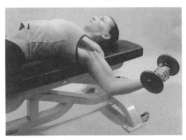

The risk is increased stress on the shoulder joint and capsule.

Incline dumbbell press *Elbows in line with the shoulders at the bottom position*

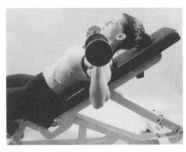
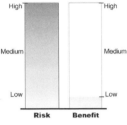

The risk is increased stress on the shoulder joint and capsule. The benefit is increased stress on the upper pectoral muscles.

Incline dumbbell press *Elbows in front of the shoulders at the bottom position*

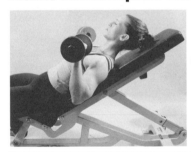
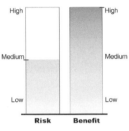

The benefit is decreased stress on the shoulder joint and capsule if the person has decreased range of motion in the shoulder. Good exercise modification when experiencing pain while performing the incline press.

Pec dec *Elbows slightly in front of shoulders at start*

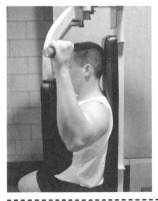
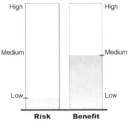
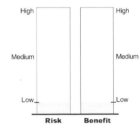

The benefit is decreased stress on the shoulder joint and capsule. The loss of benefits is decreased stress on the pectoral muscles. Good exercise modification when experiencing pain while performing the pec dec.

Pec dec *Elbows in line with shoulders at start*

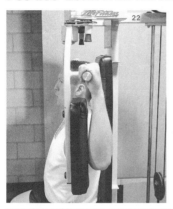

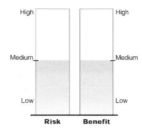

The risk is increased stress on the shoulder joint and capsule. The benefit is increased stress on the pectoral muscles for development. Most machines use this starting position.

Pec dec *Elbows behind the shoulders at start*

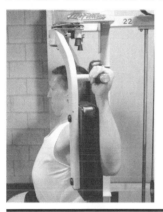

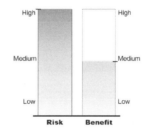

The risk is excessive stress on the shoulder joint and capsule.

Dumbbell shoulder press *Elbows in line with shoulders (at 3:00 and 9:00) in the bottom position*

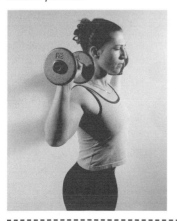

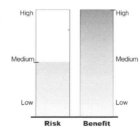

Good shoulder flexibility is needed to get the elbows back in line with the shoulders, stressing the shoulder joints and capsules. The benefit is maximal stress on all the shoulder muscles.

Dumbbell shoulder press *Elbows in front of shoulders (at 4:00 and 8:00) in the bottom position*

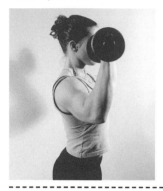

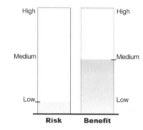

Less shoulder flexibility is needed, thus less stress is put on the shoulder joint and capsule. Less stress is put on all the shoulder muscles, and more is put on the anterior deltoid. Good exercise modification when experiencing pain while performing the dumbbell shoulder press.

Dumbbell shoulder press *Elbows in front of shoulders (at 5:00 and 7:00) in the bottom position*

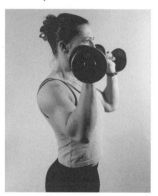

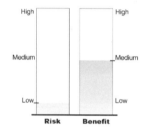

Less shoulder flexibility is needed, with less stress on the joint and capsule. Even less stress is put on all the shoulder muscles, and more is put on the anterior deltoid. Good exercise modification when experiencing pain while performing the dumbbell shoulder press.

Dumbbell shoulder press *Forward forearm angle with hands in front of elbows in the bottom position*

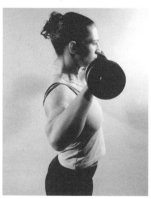

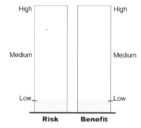

Most beginners use this position and do not keep the forearm perpendicular to the floor. The dumbbells end up too far in front of the shoulders; holding them there requires more energy.

Barbell shoulder press *Elbows in line with shoulders (at 3:00 and 9:00) in the bottom position*

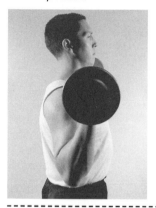

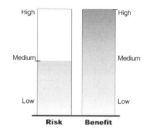

Good shoulder flexibility is needed to get the elbows back in line with the shoulders, putting stress on the shoulder joint and capsule. The benefit is maximal stress on all the shoulder muscles.

Barbell shoulder press *Elbows in front of shoulders (at 4:00 and 8:00) in the bottom position*

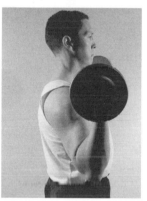

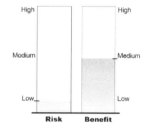

Less shoulder flexibility is needed with the elbows in front of the shoulders; thus less stress is put on the shoulder joint and capsule. Less stress is put on all the shoulder muscles, and more is put on the anterior deltoid. Good exercise modification when experiencing pain while performing the barbell shoulder press.

Barbell shoulder press *Elbows in front of shoulders (at 5:00 and 7:00) in the bottom position*

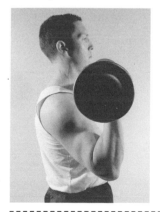

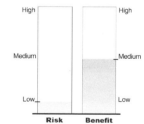

Less shoulder flexibility is needed with the elbows directly in front of the shoulders; thus less stress is put on the shoulder joint and capsule. Even less stress is put on all the shoulder muscles, and more is put on the anterior deltoid. Good exercise modification when experiencing pain while performing the barbell shoulder press.

Barbell shoulder press *Pressing the bar from behind the head*

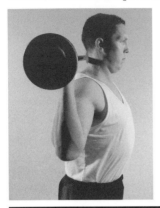

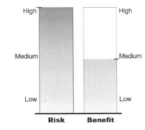

Risk   Benefit

This puts maximal stress on the cervical muscles and disks and increases risk of cervical disk herniation and stresses the shoulder capsule. The benefit is that the elbows are forced to be in line with the shoulders, which puts maximal stress on all the shoulder muscles. Excellent shoulder flexibility is needed to get the bar behind the neck.

Dumbbell lateral raise *Dumbbell in line with shoulder at the top position*

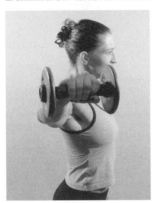

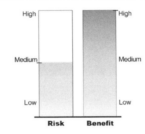

Risk   Benefit

The benefit is that maximal stress is put on the lateral deltoid muscle. Good shoulder and chest flexibility is needed to get the elbows back in line with the shoulders.

Dumbbell lateral raise *Dumbbell slightly in front of the shoulder at the top position*

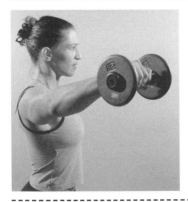

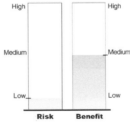

Risk   Benefit

Less shoulder and chest flexibility is needed. Less stress is put on the lateral deltoid muscle. Good exercise modification when experiencing pain while performing the lateral dumbbell raise.

Dumbbell lateral raise *Dumbbell excessively higher than the shoulder at the top position*

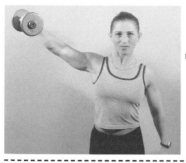

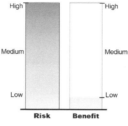

The higher the dumbbell is raised above shoulder height, the more impingement occurs in the shoulder joint.

Dumbbell lateral raise *Elbows locked during the exercise*

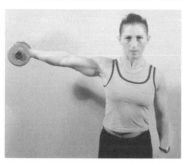

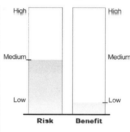

This puts more stress on the elbow joints.

Dumbbell lateral raise *Thumb rotated lower than the little finger at the top position*

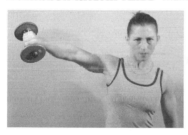

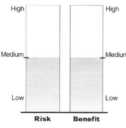

This was a very popular technique a few years ago. It can contribute to shoulder impingement when the greater tubercle of the humerus abuts the acromion. The benefit is that it potentially increases the stress on the lateral deltoid muscle.

Bent-over dumbbell lateral raise *Dumbbell in line with shoulder at the top position*

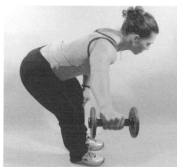

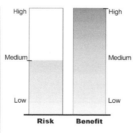

The benefit is that maximal stress is put on the posterior deltoid muscle. Good shoulder and chest flexibility is needed to get the elbows back in line with the shoulders.

Bent-over dumbbell lateral raise *Dumbbell slightly behind the shoulder at the top position*

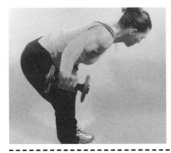

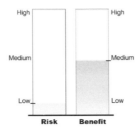

Less shoulder and chest flexibility is needed. Slightly less stress is put on the posterior deltoid muscle.

Bent-over dumbbell lateral raise *Elbows locked during the exercise*

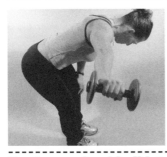

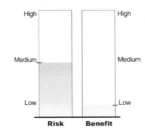

This puts more stress on the elbow joints.

Bent-over dumbbell lateral raise *Rotating the thumb lower than the little finger at the top position*

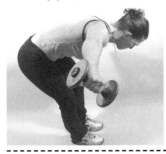

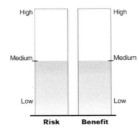

This can contribute to shoulder impingement. The benefit is that the stress on the posterior deltoid muscle increases.

Bent-over dumbbell lateral raise *Bent over 45 degrees instead of 90 degrees at the waist*

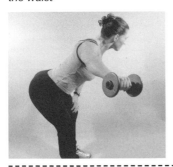

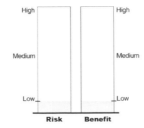

This position is not optimal to stress the posterior deltoid maximally.

Lat pulldown *Bar pulled down to the front of the neck*

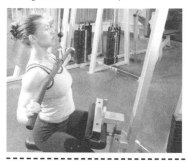

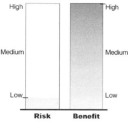

This allows full extension of the arm with maximal scapular retraction.

Lat pulldown *Bar pulled down behind the head*

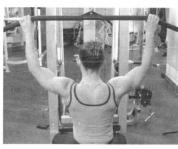

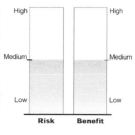

This puts increased stress on the cervical muscles and disks with increased risk of cervical disk herniation and stresses the shoulder capsule. The benefit is that the elbows are forced into line with the shoulders to put maximal stress on latissimus dorsi. Excellent shoulder flexibility is needed to get the bar behind the neck.

Lat pulldown *Bar not raised all the way up*

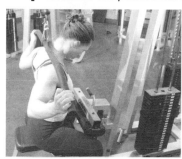

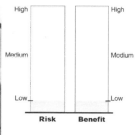

This prevents full range of motion and decreasing the stress on the latissimus dorsi. This is a common error by beginners.

One-arm dumbbell row *Upper body supported with one arm on a bench while bent over*

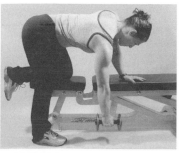

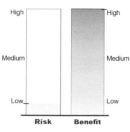

This decreases fatigue in the lower back from maintaining the bent-over posture.

One-arm dumbbell row *No support of the upper body while bent over*

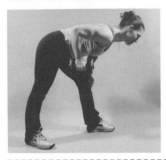

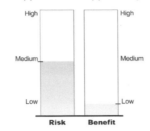

This increases the fatigue in the lower back from maintaining the bent-over posture.

One-arm dumbbell row *Not pulling the dumbbell high enough*

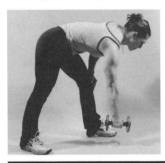

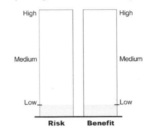

This prevents full contraction of the latissimus dorsi and rhomboid muscles.

Seated cable row *Sitting straight up at the end of the exercise; with handle in the abdominal region*

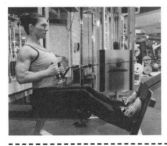

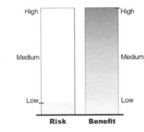

The benefit is maximal arm extension and scapular retraction for upper-back development.

Seated cable row *Excessive backward leaning at the end of the exercise with handle in the abdominal region*

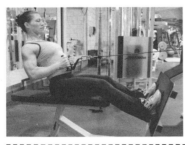

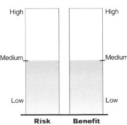

A forced back extension with weight increases the risk of lumbar facet joint irritation.

Seated cable row *Slight forward lean; starting with the handle at arms' length*

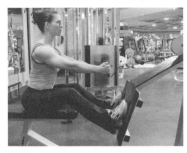

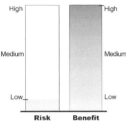

This is a good starting position with full arm extension and scapular protraction to permit full range of motion with minimal stress on the lower back.

Seated cable row *Excessive forward lean in the starting position with the handle at arms' length*

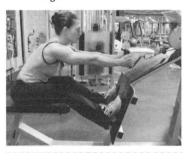

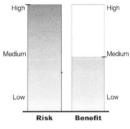

This increases the risk of lumbar disk and ligament injury due to forced flexion when using increased weight and speed.

Seated cable row *Knees slightly unlocked during the exercise*

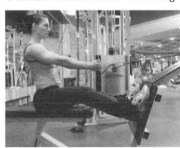

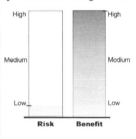

This decreases the risk of tension on the hamstrings and lower back.

Seated cable row *Knees locked during the exercise*

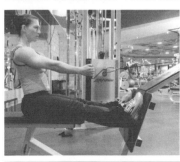

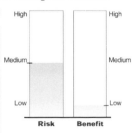

This increases the risk of tension on the hamstrings and lower back

Shrug *Head straight while moving the shoulders up and down*

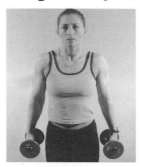

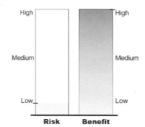

The upper trapezius is in the proper position for maximal contraction. There is no stress on the cervical muscles or disks.

Shrug *Head flexed forward while moving the shoulders up and down*

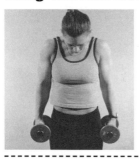

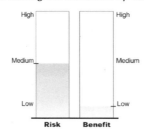

This puts stress on the cervical muscles and disks and increases the risk of cervical disk herniation.

Shrug *Head flexed forward while moving the shoulders up and down; holding breath during the set*

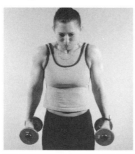

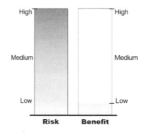

Breath holding increases interthoracic pressure, puts excessive stress on the cervical muscles and disks, and increases the risk of cervical disk herniation.

Shrug *Shoulders rolling backward on the ascent and forward on descent.*

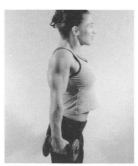

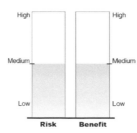

Contraction of the rhomboid and mid-trapezius muscles minimally increases when the scapulas are retracted. Increases the risk to the A/C and S/C joint.

Dead lift *Bar touches or remains within one inch of the legs while lifted*

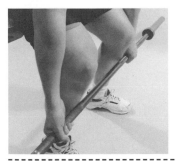

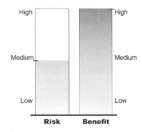

This position allows maximum leverage for strengthening all the muscles used in everyday life to lift objects off the floor.

Dead lift *Bar is within two to four inches of the legs while lifted*

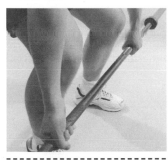

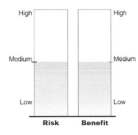

This position does not offer maximum lifting leverage. The farther the bar drifts from the body, the more force it takes to lift the bar.

Dead lift *Bar is five or more inches from the legs while lifted*

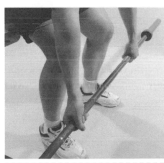

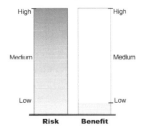

The risk of lumbar disk and ligament injury increases as the main lower-back extensor muscles are stressed maximally. The farther the bar drifts away from the body, the more force it takes to lift the bar.

Dead lift *Flat or slightly arched back maintained throughout the exercise*

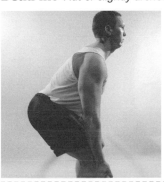

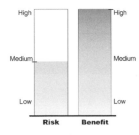

This is a good biomechanical position to lift the weight with normal stress on the disk and ligaments.

Dead lift *Starting with a flat or slightly arched back and rounding the back when the weight passes the knees*

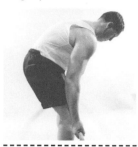

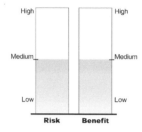

Benefit decreases due to increased stress on the vertebrae and ligaments with loss of lumbar lordosis.

Dead lift *Rounding the back throughout the entire exercise*

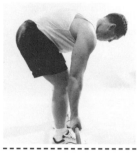

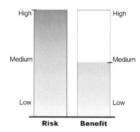

Risk increases due to maximal stress on the vertebrae and ligaments with loss of lumbar lordosis.

Dead lift *Hyperextending the back at the end of the lift*

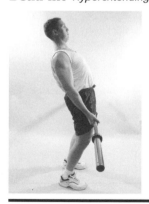

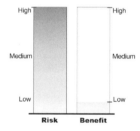

Risk increases due to lumbar facet irritation with forced lumbar extension and axial compression.

Back extension *Upper body below parallel with the floor in the end position*

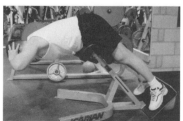

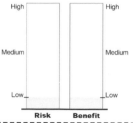

Both risk and benefit are low due to low stress on the lower back and a limited range of motion.

Back extension *Upper body parallel with the lower body in the end position*

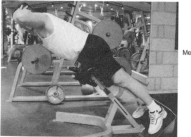

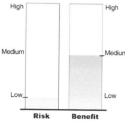

The benefit is increased stress on the lower-back muscles with the increased range of motion, which requires more back extensor muscles to contract.

Back extension *Upper body above parallel with the lower body in the end position*

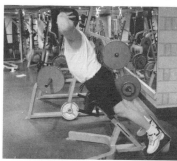

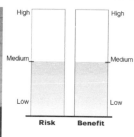

The benefit is increased stress on the lower-back muscles with the increased range of motion, which requires more back extensor muscles to contract. The risk is potential lumbar facet irritation with the hyperextension.

Back extension *The spine curled and flexed at the bottom position and slowly extended during the ascent*

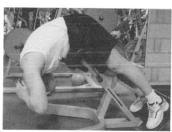

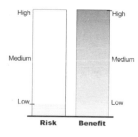

The benefit is increased stress on the lower-back muscles with the increased range of motion, which requires more intrinsic back extensor muscles to contract. Risk decreases because the spine goes through normal flexion and extension with no axial load.

Barbell curl *Full extension of arm at the start of the exercise*

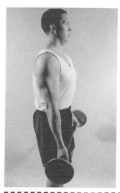

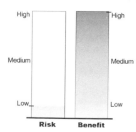

The benefit is a full range of motion will increase maximal contraction of the biceps

Barbell curl *Body sway (cheating) during the exercise*

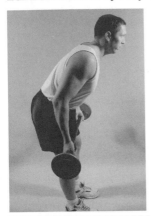

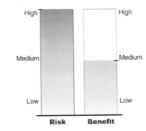

This increases the weight that can be lifted, but it also decreases the stress on the biceps. It also increases the risk of lumbar facet irritation.

Barbell curl *Wide grip*

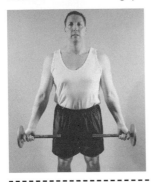

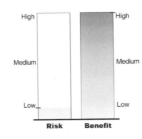

A wide grip focuses more stress on the short head (inside head) of the biceps.

Barbell curl *Narrow grip*

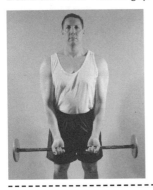

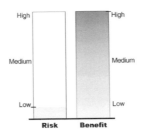

A narrow grip focuses more stress on the long head (outside head) of the biceps.

Barbell curl _Using the E-Z curl bar_

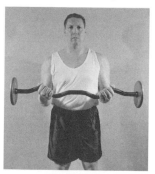

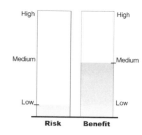

The benefit is decreased stress on the wrist, but there is also less stress on the biceps since it is involved in supination.

Alternate dumbbell curls _Full extension of arm at the start of the exercise_

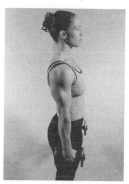

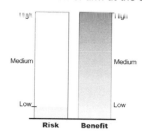

The benefit is a full range of motion will increase maximal contraction of the biceps

---

Alternate dumbbell curls _Body sway (cheating) during the exercise_

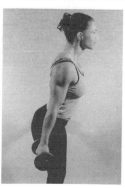

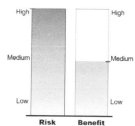

This increases the weight that can be lifted, but it also decreases the stress on the biceps. The risk of lumbar facet irritation increases.

Alternate dumbbell curls *Supination of the hand*

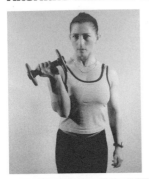

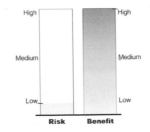

This increases activiation of the biceps since it is involved in supination. Supination is the main reason to use dumbbells instead of a barbell.

Dumbbell preacher curl *Elbows at the bottom of the pad*

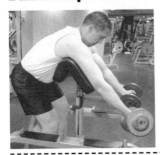

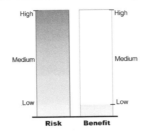

The risk of hyperextending the elbow increases. The risk of cervical disk injury also increases because the head is forward and the shoulders rounded.

Dumbbell preacher curl *Elbows at the top of the pad*

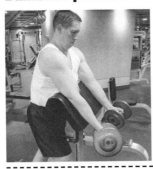

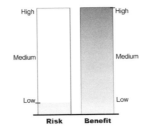

The risk of hyperextending the elbow decreases because the forearms hit the pads at normal arm extension. Chest high with the shoulders back, reduces the risk of cervical disk injury.

Dumbbell preacher curl *Stopping slightly before the forearms are perpendicular to the floor.*

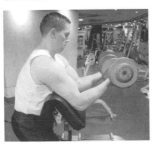

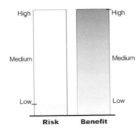

The benefit is constant stress on the biceps for maximal development.

Dumbbell preacher curl *Stopping after the forearms move slightly past perpendicular to the floor*

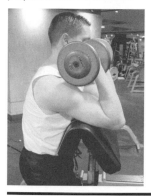

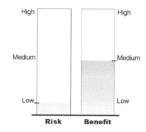

The benefit decreases because gravity takes over to help pull the dumbbells, resulting in less stress on the biceps.

Triceps push-down *Not fully extending the arm*

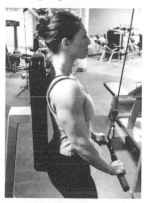

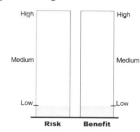

Benefit is low because triceps cannot fully contract. Common error with beginners.

Triceps push-down *Keeping the elbows tucked in beside the body during the exercise*

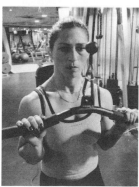

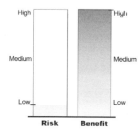

This position, known as the bodybuilding style, concentrates on the lateral triceps head but still stresses all three heads.

Triceps push-down *Allowing the elbows to swing away from the body*

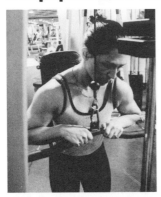

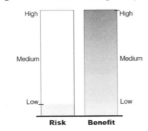

This position, known as the powerlifting style, increases the weight that can be lifted and concentrates on the long head of the triceps, which usually only works when heavy weights are lifted.

Lying triceps extension *Bringing bar to the forehead*

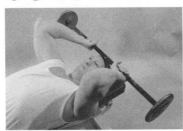

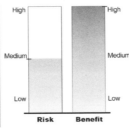

This maximizes the stress on the triceps. Stress increases on the triceps tendon where it inserts in the elbow, potentially causing pain and tendinitis.

Lying triceps extension *Bringing bar to the nose*

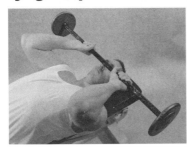

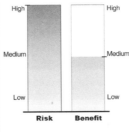

The increased angle of the elbow at the bottom position causes more stress in the elbow joint and increases the risk of facial injury if the weight slips or sudden fatigue occurs.

Lying triceps extension *Using an E-Z curl bar*

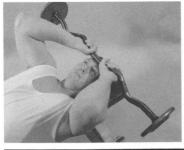

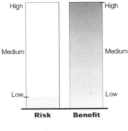

Less stress on the wrist decreases the risk of injury to the wrists.

Triceps kickback *Upper body supported with one arm on a bench while bent over*

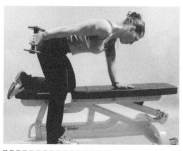

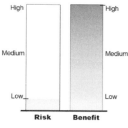

Risk decreases because the support for maintaining the bent-over posture reduces fatigue in the lower back.

Triceps kickback *No support of the upper body while bent over*

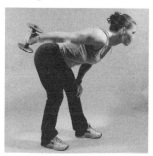

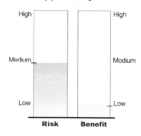

Risk increases because of fatigue in the lower back from maintaining an unsupported bent-over posture.

Triceps kickback *Not fully extending the arm*

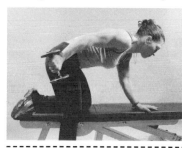

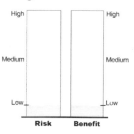

Low benefit because the triceps cannot fully contract. Common error with beginners.

Triceps kickback *Bending 45 degrees at the waist instead of 90 degrees; arm not parallel with the floor*

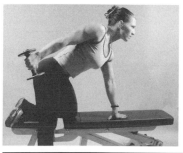

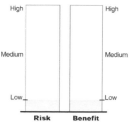

Low benefit because the triceps is not in the proper position to be stressed maximally and is using gravity to help lock it out.

Reverse curl *Using a straight bar*

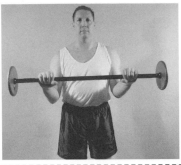

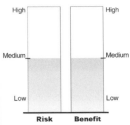

Holding the wrist in pronation increases stress on it. Increased stress on the radiobrachialis and brachialis contraction.

Reverse curl *Using an E-Z curl bar*

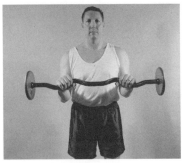

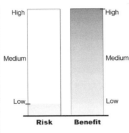

The forearm in half pronation reduces stress on the wrist and decreases risk.

Reverse curl *Starting with full arm extension*

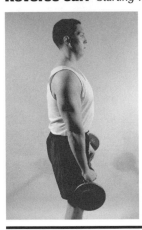

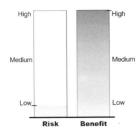

The full range of motion increases the activation of the radiobrachialis and brachialis.

Wrist extension *Decreased range of motion at the bottom position*

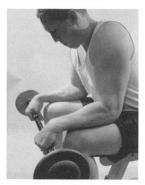

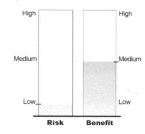

Less stress on the wrist joint decreases the risk. Full contraction of the wrist extensors offers medium benefit.

Wrist extension *Supporting the arms halfway up the forearm*

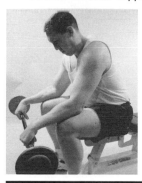

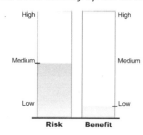

Excessive stress on the wrist joint and forearm because it is not supported.

Barbell squat *Bar carried high on the upper trapezius muscles*

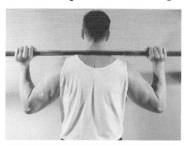

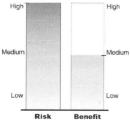

The reduced surface area for carrying the weight puts excessive pressure on the seventh cervical vertebra. The benefits are the ability to remain more upright and to stress the quadriceps muscles more.

Barbell squat *Bar carried on top of the posterior deltoids*

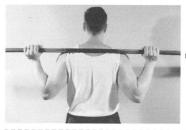

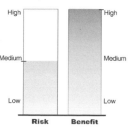

Increasing the surface area for carrying the weight puts less pressure on the cervical spine. The shorter lever arm increases potential power.

Barbell squat *Wrists hyperextended*

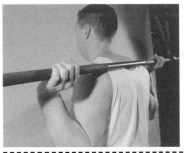

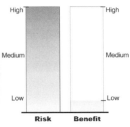

Risk | Benefit

Increased stress on the wrist joint can potentially injure the metacarpal joints in the wrist.

Barbell squat *Wrists straight*

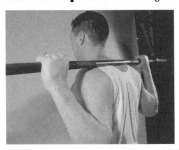

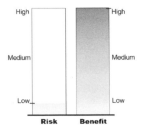

Risk | Benefit

Less stress on the wrist joint decreases risk of injury to the metacarpal joints. There is more control of the bar as it sits on the shoulders.

Barbell squat *Knees stay over the feet throughout the exercise*

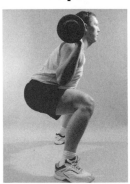

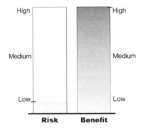

Risk | Benefit

Benefits are less stress on the knee joint and maximal leverage for power from the hip and gluteal muscles. Potentially increases stress on the lower back joints. This is known as the powerlifting style.

Barbell squat *Knees move over the feet during the exercise*

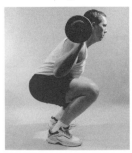

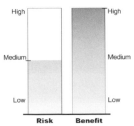

Risk | Benefit

The increased knee angle increases stress on the knee joints and ligaments. The benefit is increased stress on the quadriceps muscle. This is known as the bodybuilding style.

Barbell squat *Knees move medially to the feet (inward) during the exercise*

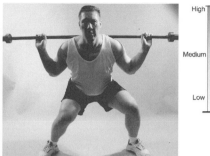

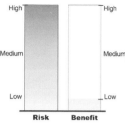

Increased stress on the knee joints and ligaments increases risk. Medial knee shift shows a potential weakness of the medial quadriceps muscles. The minimal benefit is more power from recruiting supporting muscles.

Barbell squat *Hips remain under the shoulders at the bottom of the squat during the ascent*

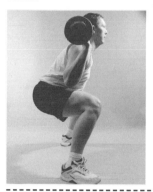

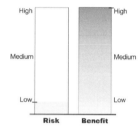

This is proper position for maximal power with decreased risk of injury to the lower back.

Barbell squat *Hips move posteriorly at the bottom of the squat during the ascent, causing the person to be bent over during ascent*

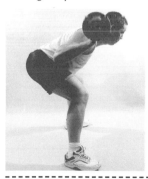

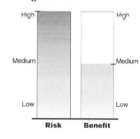

The risk is increased stress on the lower back. Common error with beginners.

Barbell squat *Shoulder-width stance*

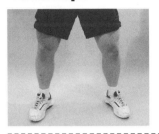

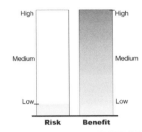

Equal amounts of stress are put on the legs, hips, and gluteal region. This is a good technique for most people.

Barbell squat *Narrow stance*

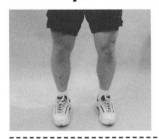

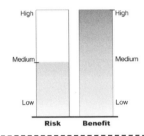

The greater knee angle increases stress on the knee joints. The benefit is a maximum stress on the quadriceps muscle.

Barbell squat *Wide stance*

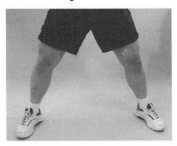

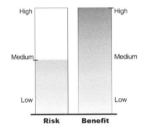

The risk is increased stress on the hip joints. The benefit is maximum stress on the hip and gluteal muscles.

Leg extension *Feet pointed straight forward*

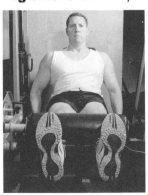

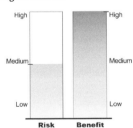

This stresses all the quadriceps muscles. The risk is some stress on the ACL ligament.

Leg extension *Feet internally rotated*

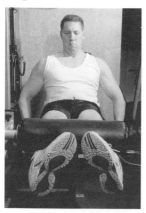

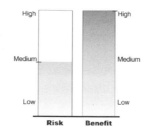

When the feet are internally rotated in (pointing the toes in), it increases the stress on the vastus lateralis for strength and development. The risk is increased stress on the knee joint as the leg goes through the extension motion while in rotation.

Leg extension *Feet externally rotated*

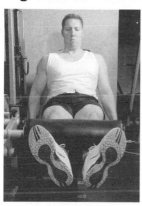

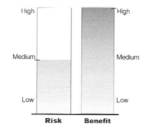

When the feet are externally rotated out (pointing the toes out), it increases the stress on the vastus medialis for strength and development. The risk is increased stress on the knee joint as the leg goes through the extension motion while in rotation.

Leg extension *Upper body tilted backward*

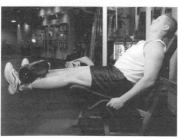

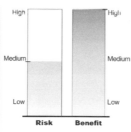

The posterior tilt of the pelvis increases the stress on the rectus femoris muscle.

Leg press *Foot platform lowered until the knee joint angle is 90 degrees*

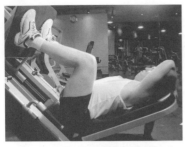

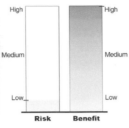

This position offers good range of motion with minimal stress on the lower back. This is a good technique for most people.

Leg press *Foot platform lowered until lumbar lordosis is diminished*

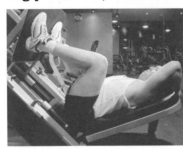

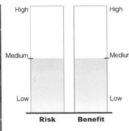

The benefit is increased range of motion and stress on the leg muscles. The risk is increased stress on the lower-back discs and joints.

Leg press *Foot platform lowered until the sacrum starts to rotate off the pad*

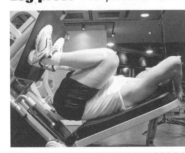

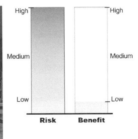

Severe stress on the lumbar ligaments and disks increases risk.

Leg press *Holding breath during the set*

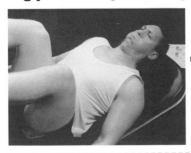

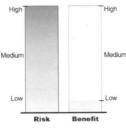

Breath holding significantly increases interthoracic pressure and the risk potential of disk herniation.

Leg press *Feet placed high on the platform*

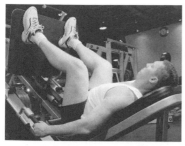

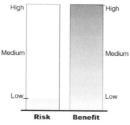

More stress is placed on the gluteals, hamstrings, and quadriceps.

Leg press *Feet placed low on the platform*

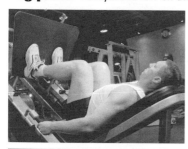

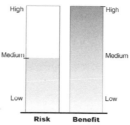

The benefit is increased stress on the quadriceps. Excessive flexion of the knee and ankle joint stress the ligaments.

Dumbbell lunge *Medium step width with knee over the ankle*

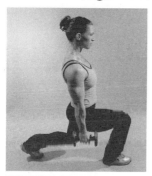

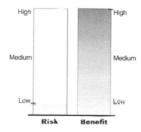

This normal range of knee motion puts stress on the quadriceps and gluteal muscles. This is a good technique for most people.

Dumbbell lunge *Long step width with knee over the ankle*

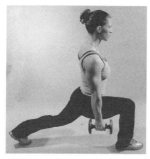

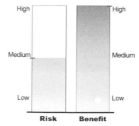

The benefit is increased stress on the gluteal and hamstring muscles. One ilium moving forward and the other backward increases risk of injury to the sacroiliac joints. This position can create or expose a sacroiliac dysfunction.

Dumbbell lunge *Short step width with knee over the ankle*

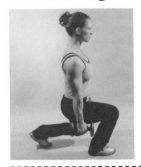

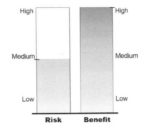

The benefit is increased stress on the quadriceps muscles. Knee hyperflexion in dynamic forward motion increases knee joint stress.

Dumbbell lunge *Focusing on one spot while doing the exercise*

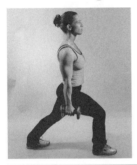

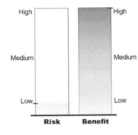

The benefit is this improves balance in dynamic motion.

Leg curl *Feet dorsiflexed*

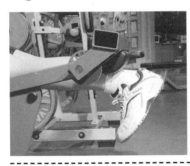

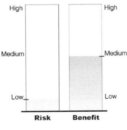

The benefit is stress on the hamstring and gastrocnemius muscle.

Leg curl *Feet plantarflexed*

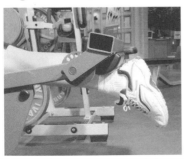

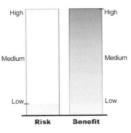

The benefit is increased stress on the hamstring with less stress on the gastrocnemius muscle.

Leg curl *Feet internally rotated*

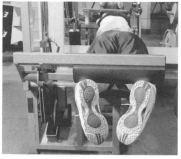

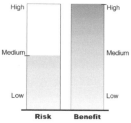

The benefit is increased stress on the biceps femoris muscle. The risk is increased stress on the knee joint when the leg flexes in the rotated position.

Leg curl *Feet externally rotated*

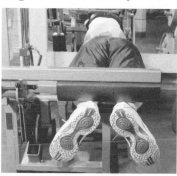

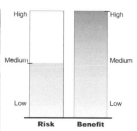

The benefit is increased stress on the semimembranosus and semitendinosus muscles. The risk is increased stress on the knee joint when leg is flexed in the rotated position.

Standing calf raise *Knees locked*

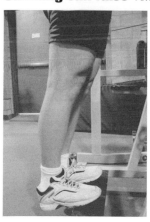

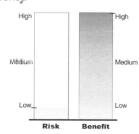

The benefit is maximal stress on the gastrocnemius muscle. This is a good technique for most people.

Standing calf raise *Hips shifting in front of shoulders during ascent*

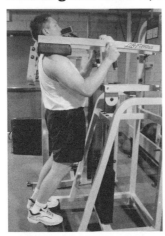

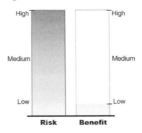

Hyperlordosis with an axial load severely increases stress on lumbar facet joints.

Standing calf raise *Neck flexed forward*

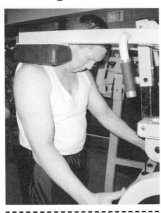

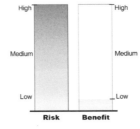

Increased stress on the cervical disk and ligaments with an axial load increases risk with no potential benefit.

Standing calf raise *Feet turned out*

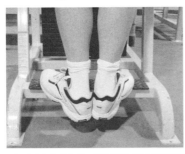

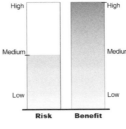

The benefit is increased stress on peroneal muscles. The risk is increased stress on the ankle joints from plantar flexion and extension with external rotation.

Standing calf raise *Feet turned in*

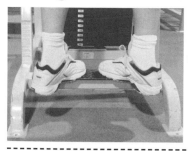
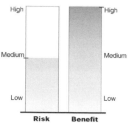

The benefit is increased stress on the posterior tibialis muscle. The risk is increased stress on the ankle joints from plantar flexion and extension with internal rotation.

Standing calf raise *Rising up on the big toe at the top of the movement*

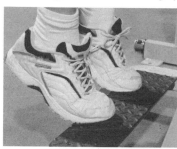
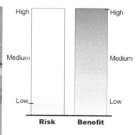

This increases the contraction of the gastrocnemius muscle and activates the flexor hallucis longus and brevis muscle, which flexes the big toe and assists in running and jumping.

Seated calf raise *Pad too far down the leg and over the top of the patella*

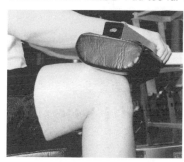
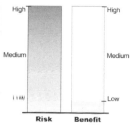

The excessive pad pressure increases the stress on the patellar tendon and bursa, potentially causing tendinitis. There is a risk of the pad slipping off the knee.

Seated calf raise *Rising up on the big toe at the top of the movement*

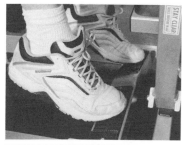
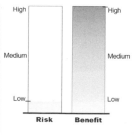

This increases the contraction of the soleus muscle and activates the flexor hallucis longus and brevis muscle, which flexes the big toe and assists in running and jumping.

Crunch *Pulling on the head while flexing the spine to contract the abdominals*

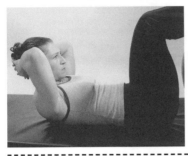

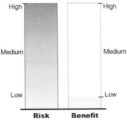

High / Medium / Low — Risk — Benefit

Excessive pulling risks injury to the cervical and thoracic muscles and ligaments.

Crunch *Holding breath during the repetition*

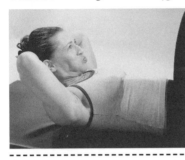

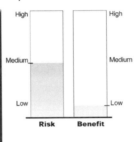

High / Medium / Low — Risk — Benefit

Breath holding causes a neurological inhibition in abdominal contraction, which decreases the benefit.

Crunch *Feet locked in under a strap or held down*

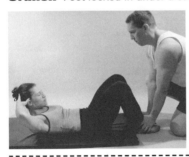

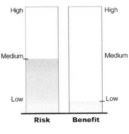

High / Medium / Low — Risk — Benefit

This decreases the benefit because it causes a neurological reflex called flexor synergy, in which recruitment of the anterior tibialis, rectus femoris, and psoas muscles which decreases the stress on the rectus abdominis.

Crunch *Touching the elbows to the knees*

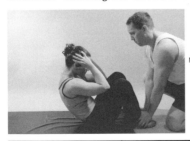

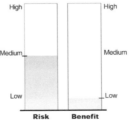

High / Medium / Low — Risk — Benefit

This decreases the benefit because the resulting trunk flexion needed to touch your elbows to your knees stresses the psoas instead of performing spinal flexion stressing the rectus abdominis.

Hanging leg raise *Legs hanging straight down at start and then flexing to 90 degrees*

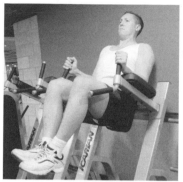

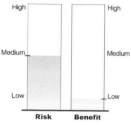

This position primarily works the psoas muscle and decreases stress on the rectus abdominis, thus decreasing the benefit to the abdominals.

Hanging leg raise *Legs flexed 90 degrees while spine curls up*

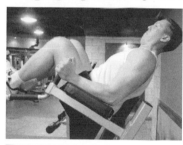

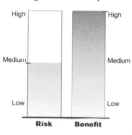

This increases the stress on the rectus abdominis and holds the psoas in a stable isometric contraction.

Summary

The application of any weight-training exercise technique depends on the outcome desired from training, whether it is strength or muscle development. The techniques in this chapter help focus maximum stress on the specifically targeted muscles while minimizing potential for injury. Let's now look at how to put these weight-training exercise techniques together into a routine to optimize strength and development.

5

Designing Training Programs for Optimal Strength

The previous four chapters offered a better understanding of how the body performs and the exercises that are most beneficial for various training outcomes and goals.

Chapter 1 revealed how the body can become dysfunctional and also offered a Weight-Training Readiness Screen and form for determining the functional level of the muscles, joints, nerves, and the body's biochemistry. This type of subjective testing, asking questions about how a person feels, determines whether there are limits to training and whether current training or treatment protocols are perceived to be beneficial.

Chapter 2 described the Weight-Training Readiness Exam, which helps determine the current state of the muscles, joints, and nervous system to reveal any hidden dysfunctions such as decreased range of motion, weakness, or pain. This type of testing, known as objective testing, determines how the body reacts to an external force and determines with greater specificity whether there is a problem and, if so, its type and severity. Objective testing allows the measurement of flexibility and strength to determine the current state and what is needed to improve function.

Chapter 3 reviewed functional anatomy, indications of weakness, optimal training principles, and how they may be applied to achieve the person's training goals.

Chapter 4 discussed the benefits and risks of various weight-training exercise techniques and how training volume and intensity is to be determined by experience level and desired outcome.

This final chapter explains how to put all this information together into a specific, individualized routine to help the person reach their optimal strength and development goals. This chapter helps determine the person's current functional ability and where the person is in their training program so he or she can reach their determined outcome of strength or development. It offers the road map to improved functional level and optimized performance.

Program Design

Designing an optimal exercise training program is a five-step process (figure 5.1). A good program design takes into consideration any obstacles to functioning that need training or treatment and simultaneously provides optimal training to look better, perform better, or both. The five steps of the process are now briefly reviewed.

Steps 1 & 2 ⟶ **Step 3**
Determine   Determine your
where you   training outcome
currently are   -Look better
                   -Perform better

Step 4-Functional training program
Step 5-Optimal training program

FIGURE 5.1   Five steps to optimal program design.

Step 1: Weight-Training Readiness Screen

The first step is determining the person's current status through the Weight-Training Readiness Screen and Weight-Training Readiness Form (forms 1.1 and 1.2) These forms reveal the functional level of specific muscles or joints and the severity of any problems in function. If the person's progress has been stalled for a period of time and the person is frequently tired, the Subjective Training Stress Level Questionnaire (form 1.3) can help determine the person's biochemical functional status.

You can access a printable version of all forms on the DVD.

Step 2: Weight-Training Readiness Exam

Next, the Weight-Training Readiness Exam, which includes a self-test, an exercise test, and a functional muscle test, should be conducted. The functional muscle test must be performed by a personal trainer, therapist, or doctor who is trained to do functional muscle testing. These tests (described in chapter 2 and demonstrated on the DVD) help determine the current state of the body and reveal any dysfunctions that may limit training.

Step 3: Determine Training Goals and Desired Outcomes

The third step is to fill out the Optimal Training Outcome and Goal Form on page 103 and on the DVD. This identifies all desired training outcomes and goals. The

Optimal Training Outcome and Goal Form

The following graphic depicts the continuum between two commonly desired training outcomes: to look better and to perform better. The desired focus on each of these outcomes varies for each person. Indicate how much focus the person wants to give each outcome. If the person wants only to look better, put 100% on the left side and fill out the appearance-related training goals completely. If the person wants only to perform better, put 100% on the right side and fill out the performance-related training goals completely. If the person wants to look and to perform better equally, put 50% on both sides and complete only one goal per training outcome (one appearance-related and one performance-related).

Training outcome   **Training outcome**

100% better appearance   50% better appearance   100% better performance

0% better performance   50% better performance   0% better appearance

_____% better appearance   _____% better performance

Goals   **Goals**

Decrease body fat   **Increase strength**

By _____ pounds   Which lifts?

In ____weeks   _____

                                                                By _____ pounds

Increase muscle mass   **Increase muscular
                                                                    endurance**

By _____ pounds   Which lifts?

In ____weeks   _____

**Focus on visually
underdeveloped body part**   How many sets
                                                                or reps? _____

❏ Shoulders

❏ Chest   **Increase sport-
                                                            specific performance**

❏ Biceps   Which sport?

❏ Triceps   _____

❏ Forearms

❏ Upper back   Which skill?

❏ Lower back   _____

❏ Thighs   How will results

❏ Calves   be measured? _____

❏ Abdominals   In _____weeks

Optimal Training Outcome and Goal Form assumes that people generally want to achieve one of three different training outcomes: to look better, to perform better in a team or individual sport or in daily life activities, or to both look and perform better.

The specific outcome that the person wants to achieve from training determines the method of training. For example, consider the squat exercise in the sports of bodybuilding and powerlifting. In bodybuilding, the goal is to look better because the person is being judged by how they look, not by how they perform. The concern is thus not with how much weight is lifted in the squat but rather with stressing the muscle maximally to induce hypertrophy. In the sport of powerlifting, the person is being judged by how they perform, not how they look. With the goal of performing better, the person does everything possible to lift more weight in the squat with little concern for how the body looks. People in these two sports use the same exercise but different techniques and intensities to achieve their desired outcomes. This illustrates why it is important to determine exactly what the person wants to accomplish, muscular hypertrophy or increased strength, to correctly design the optimal program to achieve that outcome.

The training goal of most noncompetitive weight trainers is to both look and perform better. For such people, the program design can maximize muscular gains and increase strength through periodization, emphasizing different goals in different seasons of the year (for example, focusing on strength in the fall and winter and muscle hypertrophy and definition in the spring and summer).

Once the desired training outcome is determined, some measurable goals can be set, such as target body weight, body fat, muscle changes, or strength increases in specific exercises, along with a specific timeline for them to be achieved. These goals should be set down on paper to make them more real and to provide a roadmap for getting from here to there. If goals are not written down, they tend to be forgotten and are rarely achieved.

Step 4: Design a Functional Training Program

In step 4, a functional training program is designed to improve function and correct any dysfunctions revealed in step 1 and 2. After the tests in step 2 are completed, the scoring sheets, available on the DVD, are filled out. Each of the tests has a corresponding flexibility exercise, isometric agonist-antagonist exercise, resistive tubing exercise, or active proprioceptive neuromuscular facilitation (PNF) exercise. The results from the tests determine the type of exercise to do.

Functional Training Exercises

To rebalance the body to its optimal state, four factors must be considered: range of motion, strength, pain, and coordination. Specific exercises and movements are needed to optimize these factors if they are less than optimal. This is called functional training. Functional training exercises are different from regular weight-training exercises as these exercises help correct any dysfunctions and optimize muscle, joint, and nerve function.

To increase exercise range of motion, perform the specific flexibility exercises for each weight-training exercise demonstrated on the DVD. These flexibility exercises help reestablish the normal range of motion needed to perform the weight-training exercises properly. Specific isometric agonist-antagonist, resistive tubing, and active PNF exercises are needed to strengthen muscle that may be damaged or neurologically impaired. Isometric agonist-antagonist exercises along with active PNF help reestablish the firing order to increase muscle coordination. To decrease muscle pain, first avoid the exercise that causes pain; flexibility, resistive tubing, isometric agonist-antagonist, and active PNF exercises then can help restore strength and range of motion so that the exercise in question does not cause pain anymore. If flexibility, resistive tubing, isometric agonist-antagonist, and active PNF exercises do not resolve the pain, then other types of treatment discussed in chapter 2 are needed to restore strength and range of motion.

All functional training should be done after the normal weight-training program or on a different day. The person should not do any functional exercises before heavy lifting; the person will be fatigued and weakened by functional training and the synergistic muscles may not be able to help support the heavy load of the prime movers.

Flexibility Exercises

There are many ways to stretch a muscle. The style of stretching demonstrated on the DVD is the static stretch. This common style of stretching can be done without assistance. There are more effective stretching techniques, but many of them need a partner. The static stretch technique is done by increasing the muscle and joint range of motion until resistance is felt. The person should stretch only to the point of feeling tension, not pain. If the person feels any pain, the muscle has been stretched too far and the tension on it must be reduced. The stretch is held for 10 to 15 seconds and repeated two to three times.

Isometric Agonist-Antagonist Exercises

Isometric agonist-antagonist exercise is an excellent way to reestablish the neurological firing pattern that the muscle will experience in a weight training exercise without putting the joint or muscle under a heavy dynamic load. After an injury, the nervous system receptors in the muscles, joints, ligaments, tendons, fascia, and skin are altered and may send abnormal information back to the spinal cord and brain. Two main groups of receptors are of concern here: nociceptors, or pain receptors, and mechanoreceptors, which include muscle spindles and golgi tendon organs. Nociception, or pain receptors, increases with decreased joint movement. Mechanoreceptor activity is increased with muscle contraction and joint movement and blocks nociception or pain.

When a muscle or joint is injured, movement may be decreased and abnormal, increasing the activity of nociceptors, which creates more pain in the joint. Mechanoreceptor activity is usually reduced since joint movement is restricted. Isometric agonist-antagonist exercise increases mechanoreceptor activity, which can influence the nervous system at the spinal cord level and inhibit nociceptor activity. It feels better to move an area that is injured because increased mechanoreceptor activity decreases nociception and therefore also pain.

On the DVD, there is one isometric agonist-antagonist exercise for each weight-training exercise. The isometric agonist-antagonist exercise is done by positioning the muscle and joint properly, as demonstrated on the DVD. The isometric agonist-antagonist contraction should be 60 to 80 percent of normal maximal effort and should last for eight seconds. During the first two seconds, tension is slowly increased, maximal contraction takes place during the next four seconds, and tension is slowly released in the last two seconds. Then an eight-second isometric contraction is done for the antagonist muscle, as demonstrated on the DVD. Start with one set of four to six repetitions, and add sets weekly as strength increases up to three sets. Isometric agonist-antagonist exercise helps reestablish normal neurological activity through the exercise range of motion.

Resistive Tubing Exercise

Resistive tubing exercises allow the person to move a muscle through a dynamic exercise range of motion with varying degrees of tension. For light tension at the beginning and more at the end, the exercise can begin with the tubing under minimal tension, and the tubing tension builds as the exercise movement progresses. For a lot of tension throughout the exercise, start with a lot of tension on the tubing at the beginning, and the change in tension will be minimal throughout the movement. For example, a bench press movement can start with a small amount of tension on the tubing that increases with arm extension. As the person gets stronger, the starting tension on the tubing can be increased by increasing the starting length of the tubing with only a small tension increase at the end of arm extension. This mimics free weights, since the resistance of weights does not change through the exercise movement. The benefit of tubing exercises for strengthening is that the tension can be manipulated by the type of exercise. Each weight-training exercise has a tubing exercise, demonstrated on the DVD, for rehabilitating the muscle. Start with one set of 6 to 10 repetitions, and increase by one set per week up to three sets.

Active Proprioceptive Neuromuscular Facilitation (Active PNF)

Active PNF is a combination of isometric agonist-antagonist exercise and resistive tubing exercise. The goal is to reestablish a normal neurological firing pattern through a dynamic range of motion under tension. Active PNF, demonstrated on the DVD, involves moving the arm in diagonal X pattern across the body to work various muscles and proprioceptors. This is a very effective exercise for improving the function of shoulder and chest muscles. Start with one set of 10 repetitions in both directions, and increase by one set per week up to three sets.

Step 5: Design an Optimal Training Program

In step 5, an optimal muscle training program is designed based on the desired outcome and training goals identified in step 3. The design of an optimal muscle training program must take into consideration the functional training that will be done at the end of the workout or on off days to help improve the function of specific body parts. Functional training or optimal training is done for each body part; both are done if there is a reason to, such as increasing the strength of specific synergistic muscles.

Weight Training Exercise Parameters

Designing an optimal training program must address a variety of weight-training parameters to ensure training success. The eleven different parameters are desired outcomes and training goals, exercise duration, number of training days per week, optimal time of day to train, exercise of muscle groups, muscle group priority, training equipment, accessory equipment, selection of weight-training exercises, exercise movement speed, and rest between sets.

Desired Outcomes and Training Goals

Before a person starts training, his or her desired outcomes and training goals should be determined. A desired outcome is a desired result and why it is wanted. A goal breaks up the path to achieving the outcome into small measurable steps so that progress can be measured. The most important variable in goal setting is a time frame. A specific time for reaching the outcome or result must be set.

Once the person has information about where he or she currently is on the road to optimal performance, it is time to discover where the person wants to go. As discussed in step 3, most people either want to look better or perform better in a sport or in everyday activities such as walking, running, and household chores. A few want to strengthen themselves for specific weight-training sports such as powerlifting or Olympic lifting.

Exercise Duration

In a well-designed weight-training program, the duration of exercise training should be long enough to provide optimal stimulation but not so long that energy levels and hormonal levels decrease. Russian research revealed that short-term changes in the testosterone-to-cortisol ratio reached a peak after approximately 45 minutes of heavy resistance training. For heavy strength training, shorter workouts of 20 to 40 minutes are optimal, whereas for muscular hypertrophy 30- to 60-minute workouts are optimal.

Number of Training Days per Week

The number of training days per week depends on the person's experience level, current recuperation capacity, and specific type of training (for example, high-intensity, low-volume strength work or high-volume, low-intensity muscular hypertrophy or endurance work). In general, the more intense the workout, the less frequently the person should train. For example, if the person trains at 80 to 90 percent of the one-repetition maximum (2-5 repetitions per set) training frequency can be three to four times a week. If the training intensity is 65 to 75 percent of the one-repetition maximum (8-12 repetitions per set) training frequency can be increased to four to six times a week.

Time of Day

Due to the 9–5 work schedule, most people train either at 6–7 A.M. or 6–8 P.M. and both times have their strengths and weaknesses. People who train in the morning have difficulty with the high-intensity, low-volume work needed for strength and developing the nervous system. Low-intensity, high-volume muscle hypertrophy work is easier in the morning. Nighttime can be the optimal time for high-intensity strength training or lower-intensity muscle hypertrophy training.

These two questions below can help determine the time of day when training works best for a particular person's body cycles:

1. Does the person wake up tired in the morning and need an alarm clock to get up?
2. Does the person stay up after 11:00 p.m. and feel energetic?

Answering yes to both questions identifies a night person who should train at night for optimal results. No to both means morning training may be more effective. No to question 1 and yes to question 2 means the person can train either in the morning or at night. Yes to question 1 and no to question 2 means the person may be overstressed; his or her nutrition and vitamin level need to be looked at, but night training is probably better at this time.

Muscle Group Training Combinations
The selection of muscle group training combinations depends on the training outcome wanted. The first choice is one exercise for each body part to train the whole body in one day. Another choice relies on movement patterns; the most common is the push/pull grouping, in which the chest, shoulders, and triceps are trained on one day and the legs, back, and biceps on the following day. The third grouping combines different body parts for muscle hypertrophy, for example, chest and back on one day, shoulders and arms the next day, legs on the last day. Very advanced muscle hypertrophy training can exercise one body part per day, for example, the chest on Monday, the back on Tuesday, shoulders on Wednesday, arms on Thursday, and legs on Friday, with Saturday and Sunday off. To group the exercises based on the powerlifts, do a heavy bench press with light shoulder and triceps workout on Monday, heavy squats with a light back workout on Tuesday, rest on Wednesday, a light bench press with heavy shoulder and triceps workout on Thursday, and heavy dead lifts with a light leg workout on Friday. Abdominals and calves can be exercised three to five times a week at the end of the workout.

Muscle Group Priority
Generally, the largest body parts are trained first down to the smallest body parts last. Always train the chest and shoulders before the triceps and the back before the biceps to reduce loss of arm strength in the heavy chest, shoulder, and back workout. The exception to this rule is an example when an arm muscle, such as the biceps, needs strengthening or specific focus; in that case, it should be trained first, when energy and strength are highest, to maximize muscular hypertrophy. The back should be trained on a separate day.

Training Equipment
Training equipment choices include free weights (such as barbells and dumbbells), selectorized weight machines, plate-loaded weight machines, cable machines, and equipment for body-weight exercises such as bars for chin-ups and dips. The selection of equipment depends on the desired outcome. In general, for strength training, free weights should be used predominantly, with some machine, cable, and body-weight work. In general, for muscular hypertrophy, relatively equal amounts of free-weight,

machine, cable, and body-weight exercises should be used because machines are able to isolate specific muscles more effectively than some compound free-weight exercises.

Accessory Equipment

It is important to know when to use and when not to use weight-training accessories such as wraps, straps, and weight belts. Generally, refrain from using accessories during high-volume, low-intensity training. Wrist wraps can be utilized when heavy weights are used in the following exercises: bench press, dumbbell press, squats, barbell and dumbbell curls, and any heavy Olympic lifting exercise, such as the power clean and snatch and the clean and jerk. Knee wraps can be used for heavy squats, dead lifts, and very heavy leg presses. Weight belts can increase intrathoracic pressure to help stabilize the spinal column during heavily axially loaded exercises such as the squat, dead lift, and overhead press. People should not develop the habit of wearing a weight belt tightly at all times, as this does not allow the core abdominal muscles to be exercised appropriately during general training.

Selection of Weight-Training Exercises

The selection of weight-training exercises is based on the desired training outcome. In general, it is best for beginners to use compound, multijoint exercises rather than isolated, single-joint exercises. The first six weeks of weight-training exercises develop the nervous system, especially the proprioceptive and muscular coordination of exercise movement. This development is reduced if the person uses machines that work in only one plane of motion decreasing synergistic muscle activation that may later cause potential problems when using free weights.

Generally, the person should start with a compound movement first, such as the bench press, which uses both the shoulder and elbow joints. After the bench press the person can progress to the dumbbell fly, which uses only the shoulder joint. In a advanced training technique for muscular hypertrophy called pre-exhaust training, the isolation exercise, such as the dumbbell fly, is done first and then the multijoint exercise, such as the bench press, is done afterward to use the triceps to further exhaust the pectoral muscles for more hypertrophy stress.

Exercise Movement Speed

There are four exercise movement speeds: slow, medium, fast, and explosive. Strength coaches Charles Poliquin and Ian King have both popularized different speed-of-movement training methods that use a specific amount of time for the descent, bottom position, and ascent to achieve a specific training effect. Drawing from these training concepts, slow ascents or descents should take about three seconds. Medium-speed ascents or descents should take about two seconds. Fast ascents or descents should take one second. For specific free-weight exercises such as the bench press, overhead press, squat, and dead lift, which can use an explosive ascent speed, the goal is less than one second.

In general, medium-speed ascent and descent movements are the most effective for beginners and intermediate lifters. This speed allows enough time under tension to create a muscular hypertrophy and strength response safely and effectively. For specific exercises such as the squat and bench press, competitive lifters can use a slow descent speed and fast or explosive ascent speed for increased strength.

Rest Between Sets

The length of time between sets is determined by the physiological effect of training on the body. To lift as much weight as possible, longer rest periods are needed between sets. To increase muscle hypertrophy, shorten the rest time between sets.

A bout of heavy and rapid breathing occurs immediately after an intense set. The oxygen taken into the body above normal resting oxygen consumption is used to produce extra adenosine triphosphate (ATP). Rest intervals allow the body to replenish the phosphocreatine (PC) and ATP stores for the next set and are a major source of energy for maximal lift. Studies by Diprampero and Margaria and by Meyer and Terjung found the following ATP-PC replenishment rates: Within 20 seconds of rest, 50 percent of the depleted ATP and PC is replenished. Within 40 seconds, 75 percent is replenished. Within 60 seconds, 87 percent is replenished. Within approximately three to four minutes, almost all the depleted ATP and PC intramuscular stores are replenished.

These studies indicate that a person should be ready to do another set within a minute. Other studies, however, showed that the nervous system, unlike the ATP system, can take up to three or four minutes to fully recover from a heavy set. It may therefore be beneficial to rest four minutes or more between heavy sets with few repetitions. Thus, a short rest time between sets encourages muscular development, whereas a long rest time allows the neurological system to recover to lift more weight.

To optimize the rest period, the person should consciously breathe deeply to increase oxygen uptake and produce more ATP for use in the next set. Also, walking between sets activates the lymphatic system to pump out the acids and metabolic wastes created by training for faster recovery. Walking also stimulates the mechanoreceptors in the body to decrease the nociceptor activity and may reduce any pain caused by the set.

Summary

This chapter provided information for designing training programs for optimal performance following a five-step process: identifying the person's current functional status through screens and exams, determining the desired training outcome, designing a functional training program to improve function and eliminate dysfunctions, and finally creating an optimal training program to help the person achieve his or her full training potential. Well-designed training programs allow the person to train optimally, despite any limitations or injuries. You now have the knowledge to design a complete training program for anyone of any experience level.

The ability to perform to the highest potential means more than lifting well in the gym; it also means overcoming limitations due to muscle, joint, or nerve dysfunctions. Limitations can hold a person back from his or her full lifting potential. All the tests and exercises in this book and DVD ensure that the person will be able to identify, fix, prevent, and also enhance their training capabilities to their full potential. Train hard and safe and best of luck!

Resources

Akeson, W., and D. Amiel. 1977. Collagen cross linking alterations in joint contractures. *Connective Tissue Research* 5: 15–19.

Albert, M. 1995. *Eccentric Muscle Training in Sports and Orthopaedics.* New York: Churchill Livingstone.

Alter, M. 1996. *Science of Flexibility.* Champaign, IL: Human Kinetics.

Alter, M. 1998. *Sport Stretch.* Champaign, IL: Human Kinetics.

Baechle, T., and R. Earle. 2000. *Essentials of Strength Training and Conditioning.* Champaign, IL: Human Kinetics.

Barnes, M. 1997. The basic science of myofascial release. *Journal of Bodywork and Movement Therapies* 1 (4): 24–30.

Bullock–Saxton, J., and V. Janda. 1993. Reflex activation of gluteal muscles in walking: An approach to restoration of muscle function for patients with low-back pain. *Spine* 18 (6): 704–708.

Butler, D. 1991. *Mobilisation of the Nervous System.* Toronto: Churchill Livingstone.

Chaitow, L. 2001. *Muscle Energy Techniques.* Toronto: Churchill Livingstone.

Chek, P. 2002. *CHEK Marks for Success,* Volume 2. Encinitas, CA: CHEK Institute.

Currier, D.T. 1962. Electromyographic studies of the extensor apparatus of the forearm. *Anatomical Record* 144: 373–376.

DeAndrade, J.R., C. Grant, and A.S.J. Doxon. 1965. Joint distension and reflex muscle inhibition in the knee. *Journal of Bone and Joint Surgery* 47: 313.

Delavier, F. 2001. *Strength Training Anatomy.* Champaign, IL: Human Kinetics.

Delavier, F. 2003. *Women's Strength Training Anatomy.* Champaign, IL: Human Kinetics.

Di Pasquale, M. 1997. *Amino Acids and Proteins for the Athlete: The Anabolic Edge.* Boca Raton, FL: CRC Press.

Donatelli, R. 1981. Effects of immobilization on the extensibility of periarticular connective tissue. *Journal of Orthopedic and Sports Physical Therapy* 3 (2): 67–72.

Dvorak, J., and V. Dvorak. 1990. *Manual Medicine Diagnostics.* New York: Thieme Medical Publishers.

Enoka, R. 1994. *Neuromechanical Basis of Kinesiology.* Champaign, IL: Human Kinetics.

Fuhr, A. 1997. *Activator Methods Chiropractic Technique.* New York: Mosby.

Gorman, D. 1981. *The Body Moveable.* Ontario: Ampersand Press.

Gunn, C. 1997. *The Gunn Approach to the Treatment of Chronic Pain.* Toronto: Churchill Livingstone.

Hammer, W. 1999. *Functional Soft Tissue Examination and Treatment by Manual Methods.* Gaithersburg, MD: Aspen.

Headley, B.J. 1993. Muscle inhibition. *Physical Therapy Forum,* November 1, 24–26.

Hyde T., and M. Gengenbach, eds. 1997. *Conservative Management of Sports Injuries.* New York: Lippincott, Williams & Wilkins.

Janda, V. 1978. Muscles, central nervous motor regulation and back problems. In *Neurobiologic Mechanisms in Manipulative Therapy,* ed. M. Korr, 27–41, New York: Plenum Press.

Janda, V. 1986. Muscle weakness and inhibition (pseudoparesis) in back pain syndromes. In *Modern Manual Therapy of the Vertebral Column,* ed. G.P. Grieve, 197–201, New York: Churchill–Livingston.

Janda, V. 1993. Muscle strength in relation to muscle length, pain and muscle imbalance. In *Muscle Strength,* ed. K. Harms–Rindahl, New York: Churchill–Livingston.

Johansson, H., and P. Sjolander. 1990. Neurophysiology of joints. In *Mechanics of Human Joints,* ed. E.L. Radin and V. Wright. New York: Marcel Dekker.

Jozsa, L., and P. Kannus. 1997. *Human Tendons: Anatomy, Physiology, and Pathology.* Champaign, IL: Human Kinetics.

Kelly, B., W. Kadrmas, and K. Speer. 1996. The manual muscle examination for rotator cuff strength: An electromyographic investigation. *American Journal of Sports Medicine* 24 (5): 581–588.

Kendall, F., E. McCreary, and P. Provance. 1993. *Muscles: Testing and Function.* Baltimore: Williams & Wilkins.

Kinakin, K. 1999. *First Annual International Weight-Training Injury Symposium Proceedings.* Toronto: SWIS.

Kinakin, K. 2000. *Second Annual International Weight-Training Injury Symposium Proceedings.* Toronto: SWIS.

Kinakin, K. 2001. *Third Annual International Weight-Training Injury Symposium Proceedings.* Toronto: SWIS.

Kinakin, K. 2002. *Fourth Annual International Weight-Training Injury Symposium Proceedings.* Toronto: SWIS.

King, I. 2000. *How to Write Strength Training Programs.* Australia: King Sports Publishing.

Kirkalkdy-Willis, W. 1998. *Managing Low Back Pain.* New York: Churchill Living-stone.

Kuipers, H., and H. Keizer. 1988. Overtraining in elite athletes. *Sports Medicine* 6: 79-92.

Lawson, A., and L. Calderon. 1997. Interex-aminer agreement for applied kinesiology manual muscle testing. *Perceptual Motor Skills* 84 (2): 539–46.

Leaf, D. 1995. *Applied Kinesiology Flowchart Manual.* Plymouth, MA.

Leahy, M. 1996. *Active Release Techniques: Soft-Tissue Management System for the Upper Extremity.* Colorado Springs, CO: Active Release Techniques, LLP.

Leisman, G., P. Shambaugh, and A.H. Ferentz. 1989. Somatosensory evoked potential changes during muscle testing. *International Journal of Neuroscience* 45 (1-2): 143–51.

Leisman, G., R. Zenhausern, A. Ferentz, T. Tefera, and A. Zemcov 1995. Electromyo graphic effects of fatigue and task repetition on the validity of estimates of strong and weak muscles in applied kinesiological muscle-testing procedures. *Perceptual Motor Skills* 80 (3 Pt. 1): 963–77.

Liebenson, C. 1996. *Rehabilitation of the Spine.* Baltimore: Williams & Wilkins.

MacNab, I. 1972. The mechanism of spondylogenic pain. In *Cervical Pain,* ed. C. Hirsch and Y. Zotterman, 89–95. New York: Pergamon Press.

Maffetone, P. 1999. *Complementary Sports Medicine.* Champaign, IL: Human Kinetics.

Margaria, R., P. Cerretelli, P.E. Di Prampero, C. Massari, and G. Torelli. 1963. Kinetics and mechanism of oxygen debt contraction in man. *Journal of Applied Physiology* 18: 371–377.

Margaria, R., R.D. Oliva, P.E. Di Prampero, and P. Cerretelli. 1969. Energy utilization in intermittent exercise of supramaximal intensity. *Journal of Applied Physiology* 26: 752-756.

Mattes, A. 2000. *Active Isolated Stretching: The Mattes Method.* Sarasota, FL: Aaron Mattes.

Matthews, G. 1991. *Cellular Physiology of Nerve and Muscle.* Boston: Blackwell Scientific Publications.

McComas, A. 1996. *Skeletal Muscle: Form and Function.* Champaign, IL: Human Kinetics.

McLaughlin, T. 1984. *Bench Press More Now: Breakthroughs in Biomechnics and Training Methods.* Auburn, AL: Thomas McLaughlin Publication.

Mennell, J. 1964. *Joint Pain.* Boston: Little, Brown and Company.

Mense, S., and D. Simons. 2001. *Muscle Pain: Understanding Its Nature, Diagnosis and Treatment.* New York: Lippincott, Williams & Wilkins.

Meyer, R., and R. Terjung. 1979. Differences in ammonia and adenylate metabolism in contraction in fast and slow muscle. *American Journal of Physiology* 237: C111-C118.

Meyer, R., and R. Terjung. 1980. AMP deamination and IMP reamination in working muscle. *American Journal of Physiology* 239: C32-C38.

Myers, T. 2001. *The Anatomy Trains: Myofascial Meridians for Manual and Movement Therapists.* Toronto: Churchill Livingstone.

Newton, H. 2002. *Explosive Lifting for Sports.* Champaign, IL: Human Kinetics.

Norris, C. 2000. *Back Stability.* Champaign, IL: Human Kinetics.

Paton M.E., and J.M. Brown. 1994. An electromyographic analysis of functional differentiation in human pectoralis major muscle. *Journal of Electromyography and Kinesiology* 4: 161–169.

Pecina, M., and I. Bojanic. 1993. *Overuse Injuries of the Musculoskeletal System.* Boca Raton, FL: CRC Press.

Perot, C., R. Meldener, and F. Goubel. 1991. Objective measurement of proprioceptive technique consequences on muscular maximal voluntary contraction during manual muscle testing. *Agressologie* 32 (10 Spec No): 471–4.

Poliquin, C. 1997. *The Poliquin Principles.* Napa, CA: Dayton Writers Group.

Porterfield J., and C. DeRosa. 1995. *Mechanical Neck Pain.* Toronto: W.B. Saunders Company.

Porterfield J., and C. DeRosa. 1998. *Mechanical Low Back Pain.* Toronto: W.B. Saunders Company.

Richardson, C., G. Jull, P. Hodges, and J. Hides. 1999. *Therapeutic Exercises for Spinal Segmental Stabilization in Low Back Pain.* Toronto: Churchill Livingstone.

Rydevik, B. 1991. Effects of acute, graded compression on spinal nerve root function and structure. *Spine* 16 (5): 487–493.

Sandler, D. 2003. *Weight Training Fundamentals.* Champaign, IL: Human Kinetics.

Schafer, R.C., and L.J. Faye. 1989. *Motion Palpation and Chiropractic Technique–Principles of Dynamic Chiropractic.* Huntington Beach, CA: Chiropractic Order Desk.

Schwarzenegger, A. 1987. *Encyclopedia of Modern Bodybuilding.* New York: Simon and Schuster.

Scott, L. 1991. *Loaded Guns.* Salt Lake City, UT: Larry Scott & Associates.

Siff, M. 2000. *Supertraining.* Denver, CO: Supertraining Institute.

Simon, D.G. 1993. *Referred Phenomena of Myofascial Trigger Points: New Trends in Referred Pain and Hyperalgesia.* Amsterdam: Elsevier.

Solomonow, M. 1998. The ligamento-muscular stabilizing system of the spine. *Spine* 23: 2552–2562.

Spencer, J.D., K.C. Hayes, and I.J. Alexander. 1984. Knee joint effusion and quadriceps reflex inhibition in man. *Archives of Physical Medicine and Rehabilitation* 65: 171.

Vleeming, A., and V. Mooney. 2001. *Fourth Interdisciplinary World Congress on Low Back and Pelvic Pain.* Montreal: European Conference Organizers.

Wall, E. 1992. Experimental stretch neuropathy, changes in nerve conduction under tension. *Journal of Bone and Joint Surgery* 74B: 124–129.

Walther, D. 1988. *Applied Kinesiology Synopsis.* Pueblo, CO: Systems D C.

Watkins, J. 1999. *Structure and Function of the Musculoskeletal System.* Champaign, IL: Human Kinetics.

Weintraub, W. 1999. *Tendon and Ligament Healing.* Berkeley, CA: North Atlantic Books.

Whiting, W., and R. Zernicke. 1998. *Biomechanics of Musculoskeletal Injury.* Champaign, IL: Human Kinetics.

Woo, S., and J. Buckwalter. 1988. *Injury and Repair of the Musculoskeletal Soft Tissues.* Park Ridge, IL: AAOS.

Yessis, M. 1992. *Kinesiology of Exercise.* Indianapolis, IN: McGraw-Hill/Contemporary Books.

Yoshitsugu, T., K. Shinji, E. Kenji, M. Tetsuya, and S. Takahiro. 2002. The most effective exercise for strengthening the supraspinatus muscle: Evaluation by magnetic resonance imaging. *American Journal of Sports Medicine* 30 (3): 374–381.

Index

Note: The italicized *f* following page numbers refers to figures.

About the Author

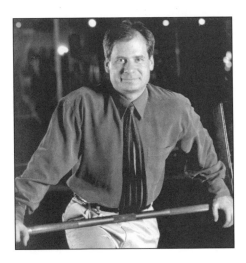

Ken Kinakin is a chiropractor, certified strength and conditioning specialist, and certified personal trainer. He has competed in bodybuilding and powerlifting for more than 20 years. He regularly lectures in Canada and the United States to doctors, therapists, and personal trainers on weight training, injury treatment, rehabilitation, and nutrition. Kinakin is on the Canadian and International Powerlifting Medical Committees. He maintains a private practice in Mississauga, Ontario, where he treats weight-training enthusiasts including Olympic and world champion athletes. Kinakin is founder and president of the Society of Wellness Integrated Specialists (SWIS), an organization dedicated to the education and training of health and fitness specialists.

OptimalMuscleTraining.com

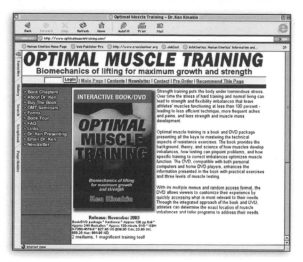

As a buyer of *Optimal Muscle Training,* you now have access to the members only section on Dr. Ken Kinakin's Web site www.OptimalMuscleTraining.com. In this section, you will find the following bonus materials:

- Written descriptions and pictures of over 200 flexibility, isometric, and tubing exercises
- Printable versions of all of the forms described in the book and on the DVD
- An in-depth review of effective treatments for weight training dysfunctions including pictures of the treatment and equipment discussed in the book along with supporting web site addresses
- Additional chapters on rest and recovery techniques
- A review of the resources used to create the book including purchase order information
- Information on Dr. Ken Kinakin's upcoming seminars and workshops

To access the members only section, go to www.OptimalMuscleTraining.com and enter the password 4679-8 into the login section.

More Muscle, More Power!

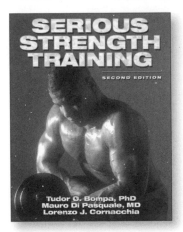

Boost your workouts and results to the next level with *Serious Strength Training!* Armed with solid scientific principles and proven training and nutrition programs, you will gain more muscle strength, mass, and definition than ever before.

From the 66 maximum muscle-stimulating exercises to the detailed dietary plans, make *Serious Strength Training* your guide to the greatest training you've ever done.

304 pages • ISBN 0-7360-4266-0

Include the snatch, clean, jerk, and their variations in your sports training program. *Explosive Lifting for Sports* and the *Explosive Lifting for Sports Video* take an in-depth look at the safest, most effective learning progressions for these lifts. With step-by-step instructions and accompanying visuals you'll see exactly how to develop the whole-body power you need to excel in your sport.

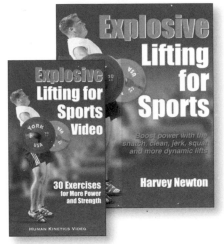

2335